CW00957312

ESSENTIAL
CLINICAL
SKILLS
FOR NURSES

⑨SAGE | 5

YEA

SAGE was founded in 1965 by Sara Miller McCune
support the dissemination of usable knowledge by publish
innovative and high-quality research and teaching conte
Today, we publish more than 750 journals, including the
of more than 300 learned societies, more than 800 n
books per year, and a growing range of library produ
including archives, data, case studies, reports, conferer
highlights, and video. SAGE remains majority-owned by
founder, and after Sara's lifetime will become owned b
charitable trust that secures our continued independen

Los Angeles | London | Washington DC | New Delhi | Singap

ESSENTIAL CLINICAL SKILLS FOR NURSES

STEP BY STEP

EDITED BY
CATHERINE DELVES-YATES

ADVISORY EDITORS:
FIONA EVERETT AND WENDY WRIGHT

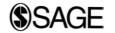

Los Angeles | London | New Delhi
Singapore | Washington DC

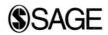

Los Angeles | London | New Delhi
Singapore | Washington DC

SAGE Publications Ltd
1 Oliver's Yard
55 City Road
London EC1Y 1SP

SAGE Publications Inc.
2455 Teller Road
Thousand Oaks, California 91320

SAGE Publications India Pvt Ltd
B 1/I 1 Mohan Cooperative Industrial Area
Mathura Road
New Delhi 110 044

SAGE Publications Asia-Pacific Pte Ltd
3 Church Street
#10-04 Samsung Hub
Singapore 049483

Editor: Becky Taylor
Development editor: Robin Lupton
Production editor: Katie Forsythe
Proofreader: Sarah Cooke
Marketing manager: Tamara Navaratnam
Cover design: Wendy Scott
Typeset by: C&M Digitals (P) Ltd, Chennai, India
Printed in Great Britain by Ashford Colour Press Ltd.

MIX
Paper from
responsible sources
FSC
www.fsc.org   FSC® C011748

Editorial arrangement © Catherine Delves-Yate

Infection and Prevention Control © Rose Gall
Clinical Measurement © Valerie Foley
Pain Management © Ann Kettyle
Aseptic Technique and Specimen Collection
Rose Gallagher
Skin Integrity © Irene Anderson and Catherin
Delves-Yates
Safer Handling of People © Dianne Steele
First Aid © Chris Mulryan and Catherine Delve.
Medicines Administration © Carol Hall and
Catherine Delves-Yates
Assisting Patients with their Nutritional Need
Kate Goodhand and Jane Ewen
Assisting Patients with their Elimination Need
Mairead Collie, David J. Hunter and Valerie F
Assisting Patients with their Hygiene Needs
Catherine Delves-Yates
Performing Last Offices © Jean Shapcott

This edition first published 2015

Apart from any fair dealing for the purposes
research or private study, or criticism or revie
permitted under the Copyright, Designs and
Patents Act, 1988, this publication may be
reproduced, stored or transmitted in any form
any means, only with the prior permission in
of the publishers, or in the case of reprograph
reproduction, in accordance with the terms of
licences issued by the Copyright Licensing A
Enquiries concerning reproduction outside th
terms should be sent to the publishers.

Library of Congress Control Number: 20149

British Library Cataloguing in Publication

A catalogue record for this book is available
the British Library

ISBN 978-1-4739-1398-1

At SAGE we take sustainability seriously. Most of our products are printed in the UK using FSC
papers and boards. When we print overseas we ensure sustainable papers are used as measured by
the Egmont grading system. We undertake an annual audit to monitor our sustainability.

CONTENTS

Assisting Patients with their Elimination Needs **129**
Mairead Collie, David J. Hunter and Valerie Foley

Assisting Patients with their Hygiene Needs **143**
Catherine Delves-Yates

Performing Last Offices **167**
Jean Shapcott

Wendy Wright and Fiona Everett

Wendy Wright and Fiona Everett

COMMON ABBREVIATIONS

Please note you may see the following abbreviations in practice. However, it is best practice to always use the full correct term to prevent mistakes and misunderstandings and to ensure patient safety.

ABG	Arterial Blood Gas
AF	Arterial fibrillation
BP	Blood pressure
C&S/ MC&S	Culture and sensitivity
CCU	Cardiac care unit / Coronary care unit
CPR	Cardiopulmonary resuscitation
CSU	Catheter specimen
CXR	Chest x-ray
DOB	Date of birth
DVT	Deep vein thrombosis
ECG	Electrocardiogram
EUA	Examination under anaesthetic
FBC	Full blood count
FBS	Fasting blood sugar
GI	Gastrointestinal
IM	Intramuscular
IV	Intravenous
KVO	Keep vein open
MI	Myocardial infarction
MRI	Magnetic resonance imaging
MRSA	Meticillin-resistant Staphylococcus aureus
MSSU/MSU	Midstream specimen of urine
NAD	No abnormalities detected
NIDDM	Non insulin-dependent diabetes mellitus
NKA	No known allergies
NOK	Next of kin

NSAID	Non-steroidal anti-inflammatory drug
O_2	Oxygen
OT	Occupational therapist
SOB	Short of breath
PR	Per rectum
PRN	Pro re nata (when required)
PUO	Pyrexia of unknown origin
PV	Per vagina
SC	Subcutaneous
TIA	Transient ischemic attack
TPR	Temperature, pulse, respiration
VS	Vital signs

USEFUL PREFIXES AND SUFFIXES

A e.g. asystole	Not, without, less
Ab, Abs e.g. abduction	From, away from
Ad e.g. adduction	Toward, in the direction of
Ambi e.g. ambidextrous	On both sides
Angi(o) e.g. angioplasty	Vessel
Ante e.g. antecedent	Before
Anti e.g. antibody	Against, opposing
Arteri(o) e.g. arteriosclerosis	Artery
Arthr(o) e.g. arthroplasty	Joint, articulation
Bi e.g. bilateral	Twice, double
Brady e.g. bradycardia	Slow
Bronch e.g. bronchitis	Bronchus
Cardio e.g. cardiomyopathy	Heart
Co e.g. comorbidity	With, together, in association with
Derm/derma/dermato e.g. dermatology	Skin
Di e.g. dissect	Separation, taking apart
Dys e.g. dysphagia	Bad, difficult
Gastro e.g. gastroenteritis	Stomach, belly
Haemo e.g. haemotology	Blood
Hyper e.g. hyperactive	Above, excessive
Hypo e.g. hypoactive	Below, deficient
Opthalm(o) e.g. ophthalmology	Eye
Pharmaco e.g. pharmacology	Drug, medicine
Phleb(o) e.g. phlebotomy	Vein
Pneum(o) e.g. pneumothorax	Air, gas, lung, breathing
Poly e.g. polycystic	Many, multiple
Tachy e.g. tachycardia	Rapid
Therm(o) e.g. thermostatic	Heat
Thora/thorac(i) e.g. thoracentesis	Chest, thorax
Uni e.g. unilateral	One, single

INFECTION AND PREVENTION CONTROL

ROSE GALLAGHER

Hand-washing

☑ **Before you start**

Consider whether it is appropriate to inform the patient that you intend to wash your hands, so the patient and their relatives or carers are reassured that you are taking steps to protect them from the transmission of infection via hands.

☑ **Essential equipment**

Running tepid water, soap, hand towels (preferably disposable, but patients may offer you a clean hand towel in community settings).

☑ **Field-specific considerations**

Washing your hands is an essential skill within the care of patients from all fields. The principles outlined in this skill will not vary depending upon field.

☑ **Care-setting considerations**

Facilities for hand-washing will vary considerably between care settings and in patients' homes.

Always be prepared for a lack of running water, soap and clean hand towels.

In community settings carry your own supply of hand towels or hand wipes to support hand-washing. Always carry hand sanitizer for situations when this is appropriate.

Keep hand sanitizers out of the reach of children or those with impaired mental capacity.

☑ **What to watch out for and action to take**

Do not apply soap directly to dry hands as this can result in sore hands and poor coverage of soap.

Staff with broken skin should cover it with a plaster. Staff unable to perform hand hygiene (because of sore hands) should not be working in clinical environments due to the risks to patients and themselves. Staff suffering from dermatitis and/or sore hands should seek advice from their local occupational health department.

Always use the foot pedal of the bin (if available) – never dispose of hand towels by lifting the lid using your fingers because this will result in recontamination of your hands.

Step	Reason and patient-centred care considerations
1. Identify the need for hand hygiene to be performed.	Undertake an assessment to ascertain whether there is a need for hand-washing to take place.
2. Turn on taps and select a comfortable temperature.	Water that is too hot or cold can impact on compliance with hand-washing technique.
3. Wet hands.	Prepares hands to receive soap and facilitates an even covering of soap for the next stage.
4. Apply soap.	Apply one dose of liquid soap to cupped hands. If bar soap is the only option available then this may be used, depending on its quality. Community staff may carry small amounts of soap with them in containers.
5. Rub hands together and evenly distribute soap coverage. (Follow the steps set out in Appendix 4, p. 190.)	Rubbing hands together produces mechanical friction. This results in all areas of the hands coming into contact with soap and transient micro-organisms being lifted from the outer layers of the skin into the soap solution on the hands.

Step	Reason and patient-centred care considerations
6. Rinse hands.	To remove the transient micro-organisms now present in the soap solution from the hands.
7. Dry hands.	Dries the skin of the hands and removes any remaining transient organisms as a result of mechanical friction. Ensure all areas of the hands are dry.
8. Dispose of hand towels.	Dispose of used materials correctly without re-contaminating your hands.

Evidence base: Loveday et al. (2013); NICE (2012a)

Using hand sanitizer

☑ **Before you start**
Consider whether it is appropriate to inform the patient that you are going to use sanitizer on your hands so the patient and their relatives or carers are reassured that you are taking steps to protect them from the transmission of infection via hands.

☑ **Essential equipment**
Hand sanitizer (this may be carried personally, available at the point of care or wall-mounted)

☑ **Field-specific considerations**
Ensuring your hands are free from transient micro-organisms is an essential skill within the care of patients from all fields. The steps outlined in this skill will not vary depending upon field.

☑ **Care-setting considerations**
Facilities for hand hygiene will vary considerably between care settings and in patients' homes.

Always be prepared for lack of running water, soap and clean hand towels. In community settings carry your own supply of hand towels or hand wipes to support hand hygiene. Always carry hand sanitizer for situations in which this is appropriate.

Keep hand sanitizers out of reach of children or those with impaired mental capacity.

☑ **What to watch out for and action to take**

Any cuts, open wounds or dry skin on hands will sting following application of hand sanitizer. Staff with broken skin should cover it with a plaster. Staff unable to perform hand hygiene (because of sore hands) should not be working in clinical environments due to the risks to patients and themselves. Staff suffering from dermatitis and/or sore hands should seek advice from their local occupational health department.

Step	Reason and patient-centred care considerations
1. Identify the requirement for hand hygiene to be performed.	Assess whether hand hygiene needs to take place. The decision to use sanitizer will depend upon being: • confident that the hand sanitizer will be effective to decontaminate hands. Remember, if a patient has diarrhoea or a gastrointestinal infection such as *C. difficile*, hand sanitizer may not be effective. Wash hands first, if possible, then apply hand sanitizer if needed. Visibly soiled hands should be cleaned with soap and water, if available, or a hand wipe prior to application of sanitizer. • able to access hand sanitizer at the point and time of need.
2. Apply the hand sanitizer to all surfaces of the hands and rub hands together to support evaporation. (See also Appendix 4, p. 190.)	All surfaces of the hands come in to contact with the hand sanitizer to ensure transient micro-organisms are destroyed.
3. Allow the hand sanitizer sufficient time to dry (evaporate) prior to next patient contact.	The hand sanitizer needs adequate time to be effective and destroy micro-organisms on hands.

Evidence base: Loveday et al. (2013); NICE (2012a)

When to remove your gloves and why

☑ **Before you start**

Ensure you have undertaken an assessment to determine if gloves can be retained or should be changed.

☑ **Essential equipment**

Hand hygiene equipment (soap and water or hand sanitizer)

☑ **Field-specific considerations**

Mental health – gloves are infrequently used in mental health settings but may be required at times. Indications may include caring for incontinent patients, phlebotomy or dressing wounds. Differences may also be present in practice depending on whether you are working in an inpatient or community setting.

Learning disability – depending on the patients, glove-use need will vary. For those with physical needs the indications for glove use are the same as for adult general nursing.

Child – indications for glove use in children's settings are the same as for adults, and this includes neonates. Newborn babies may look 'clean' but the same principles apply.

When to change gloves	Reason and patient-centred care considerations
When there is an indication for hand hygiene.	Wearing gloves may afford you some protection but the patient remains vulnerable if you do not consider the risk of transfer of micro-organisms via gloves in the same way as hands. Whenever an indication for hand hygiene occurs, and gloves are being worn, these should be removed, hand hygiene performed and then clean gloves applied. This is particularly relevant when multiple care activities are undertaken on the same patient.
When glove integrity is breached or suspected.	Gloves are not a complete barrier and defects may be present unknown to the wearer. Gloves reduce but do not eliminate risks.
When a. the actual or potential contact with blood, body fluids or mucous membranes is finished. b. contact with hazardous drugs or chemicals has finished. c. contact with a contaminated body site or device (e.g. infected wound, urinary catheter bag) has finished.	Once the activity is complete, gloves should be removed, disposed of and hand hygiene performed. This removes potential contamination from the hands of the nurse protecting both them and the next patient.

Evidence base: Loveday et al. (2013); NICE (2012a); RCN (2012)

CLINICAL MEASUREMENT

VALERIE FOLEY

Common steps for all clinical measurements

☑ **Essential equipment**

Depends upon skill but is likely to include one or more of the following:

alcohol hand-rub

fob watch with a second hand

automated non-invasive blood pressure (NIBP) machine with oxygen saturation recording device (SpO_2), or a separate oxygen saturation recording device can be used

aneroid sphygmomanometer with stethoscope

thermometer (type depends on site to be used)

blood glucose monitor and test strips

clinical waste bag

☑ **Field-specific considerations**

When caring for a patient with a learning disability it is important to know their level of understanding so that consent for and cooperation with the measurement can be gained. You will need to allow time to explain why you are doing the measurements and whether they will cause discomfort or pain.

Patients who have mental health problems or those with a learning disability may not understand the relevance of why you need to take clinical measurements. They may therefore withhold consent to have their measurements taken and you may need to refer to the Mental Capacity Act 2005 and best interest.

Children's anatomy and physiology differs to adults' and varies from birth through to adolescence. You will need knowledge of paediatric anatomy and physiology to enable you to interpret the results. As younger children do not understand why you need to take measurements, this will determine your approach to taking the clinical measurements. It is usually helpful to have the parents or carers present to assist.

☑ Care-setting considerations
It is not always possible to have all the monitoring equipment available to undertake clinical measurements. For example, in a patient's home you may not have a sphygmomanometer with stethoscope and oxygen saturation probe; however, you can still monitor the patient's respiratory rate, heart rate and capillary refill time, which will give you a clear indication of the patient's physiological condition.

☑ What to watch out for and action to take
Whilst monitoring a patient's clinical measurements you should also observe and assess:

- the colour of the skin, lips and nail beds for signs of cyanosis;
- the position of the patient;
- their neurological condition – are they alert and responsive?
- any signs or complaints of pain or discomfort;
- the patient's or relatives' views – for example saying that their condition is 'not quite right' or they 'don't feel well'.

The information gained from these observations is additional to clinical measurements and will enable you to fully assess the patient's physiological condition, institute appropriate treatment as necessary and inform senior nurses and the medical team of the patient's escalated care needs.

☑ Helpful hints – do I…?
- Gloves and aprons must be worn if contact with blood/body fluids/excreta is anticipated or the patient is in isolation.
- Hand hygiene must be performed before touching a patient, before clean/ aseptic procedures, after body fluid exposure/risk, after touching a patient and after touching a patient's surroundings.
- Waste should be disposed of in a clinical waste bag if it is contaminated with blood/body fluids/excreta.
- Equipment must be cleaned as identified by the relevant policy every time it is used.

Step	Reason and patient-centred care considerations
1. The first step of any procedure is to introduce yourself to the patient, explain the procedure and gain their consent.	Fully informed consent may not always be possible if the patient is a child, has mental health problems or has learning disabilities; even in these circumstances, however, every effort should be made to explain the procedure in terms that the patient can understand. This is not only respectful of their individual human rights, but also helps to ensure that they will be more accepting of the treatment and that their anxieties are reduced. In the case of patients who are unable to provide consent because they are unconscious, advice should be sought from your mentor or another registered nurse.
2. Gather the equipment required (see individual skills for equipment required). Ensure these are clean and in working order.	Reduces the chance of abnormal readings. Reduces the chance of infection and maintains patient and nurse safety.
3. Clear sufficient space within the environment, for example around the bed space or chair.	Enables clear access for the patient and the nurse to safely use the equipment required.
4. Wash your hands with soap and water before you start clinical measurements. If undertaking vital sign recordings on more than one patient use alcohol hand-rub between patients. Apron and gloves should only be worn if appropriate.	Wearing an apron and gloves as part of personal protective equipment (PPE) is a standard infection-control procedure when dealing with body fluids or patients in isolation. Ensure your use of PPE such as gloves and disposable aprons is appropriate by considering the individual patient situation and the risk presented.
5. Ask the patient if they wish to have the curtains drawn for privacy or to be in a separate room.	Some patients feel exposed having their clinical measurements taken in front of other people. Maintain patient privacy, dignity and comfort as required.

Step	Reason and patient-centred care considerations
6. Patients need to be in a comfortable position, either sitting in a chair, resting on a couch or in bed, unless in an emergency situation. In the case of a patient being found collapsed or acutely unwell then vital sign observations should be taken wherever the patient is situated.	To promote patient comfort and reduce anxiety.
7. If possible the patient should refrain from physical activity for 20 minutes prior to taking measurements.	Strenuous activity can falsely elevate readings.
8. Turn the monitoring equipment on and wait for it to go through its calibration checks.	Otherwise the results may be inaccurate.
9. After performing the clinical measurements, ensure the patient is in a comfortable position, with drinks and call bells available as necessary.	Promotes patient comfort and ensures they are well nourished and hydrated.
10. Discard PPE, any single-use equipment and other used materials as per policy. Clean any monitoring equipment used as per the relevant policy and perform hand hygiene.	To prevent cross-infection and maintain equipment in working condition.
11. Document findings on the patient's observation chart and/or in the patient's notes immediately.	Maintains patient safety and accurate records.
12. If any abnormal readings are observed, escalate to senior nursing staff/mentor immediately.	It is vital to report abnormal findings to a registered nurse immediately so they can ensure care is escalated. Failure to do so can result in the patient's condition deteriorating, potentially leading to death.

Evidence base: Dougherty and Lister (2011); Smith and Roberts (2011); NICE (2014a); Smith (2012); WHO (2009)

Counting a respiratory rate (RR)

☑ **What is normal?**
- Adult range: 12–18 breaths per minute (bpm)
- Child
  - Infant (birth to 1 year) 30–60bpm
  - Toddler (over 1 year to 3 years) 24–40bpm
  - Preschool (over 3 years to 5 years) 22–34bpm
  - School-aged children (over 5 years to 15 years) 18–30bpm
  - Adolescents (over 15 years to 17 years) 12–16bpm

☑ **Before you start**
Remember the common steps for all clinical measurements (pp. 8–9).

Other factors need to be considered when assessing a patient's respiratory function as it is not just the respiratory rate that detects abnormalities in breathing. As you approach the patient, observe for signs of hypoxia (severe lack of oxygen) by observing for central cyanosis (a blue/purple tint around the lips, earlobes, nose and upper chest). Does the patient appear to be breathing fast or slow, are they making any noises when breathing in or out and does it look as though their breathing is laboured?

☑ **Essential equipment**
Fob watch

☑ **Care-setting considerations**
Respiratory rates can be counted in any care setting, as long as the patient has not recently exercised and is not distressed or anxious.

☑ **What to watch out for and action to take**
If an abnormal respiratory rate is counted or any abnormalities in the respiratory function are observed this must be reported to a qualified nurse immediately and recorded in the patient's notes.

Abnormal respiratory rates can sometimes be simply improved by altering the patient's position, ensuring they have adequate analgesia or increasing the amount of oxygen being administered to the patient. However, abnormal respiratory rates must always be reported and acted upon as they can be an early sign of a patient's physiological deterioration.

Step	Reason and patient-centred care considerations
1. Perform steps 1-7 of the common steps (see pp. 8-9).	To prepare the patient and yourself to undertake the skill.
2. Ask the patient to try and remain as quiet as possible - no moving or talking. Hold their wrist as though taking their pulse.	To enable you to accurately count the respiratory rate, as talking and movement can alter the rate and make it difficult to count. By holding the wrist the patient is less likely to be aware that you are counting their respiratory rate and will not alter their pattern of breathing whilst under observation. Monitoring of a patient's respiratory rate and pulse is usually undertaken concurrently. (see p. 15).
3. Observe the patient's chest closely; count the number of breaths over one minute (60 secs) by watching the rise and fall of the chest. Each rise and fall of the chest counts as one respiration.	To obtain an accurate rate and to monitor the pattern. Respirations should always be counted for a full minute to provide an accurate recording. For example, if patients have irregular respirations, counting for less than this will produce an inaccurate value.
4. At the same time as counting the respiratory rate, note the depth of the respirations. Are they deep or shallow?	The depth of expansion of the chest gives an indication of the volume of air exchanged in each breath, which is known as the tidal volume. Shallow breathing is normally associated with a fast respiratory rate and can indicate a deteriorating respiratory condition, especially if the patient is at rest. Deep breathing may indicate a decreased level of consciousness.
5. Is the breathing pattern regular?	Irregular breathing patterns can indicate a neurological problem or be secondary to respiratory dysfunction.
6. Does the chest rise and fall equally on both sides (symmetry)?	If only one side of the chest is moving the patient may have a pneumothorax, consolidation or collapse, a mucus plug or pleural fluid in one lung.

Step	Reason and patient-centred care considerations
7. Is the patient using any accessory muscles, such as shoulders and abdominals?	Use of the accessory muscles is a sign that breathing is compromised, as they are not used in normal breathing. When pulmonary disease increases the work of breathing, the accessory muscles may be required to supplement the actions of the diaphragm and the external intercostal muscles.
8. Perform steps 9-12 of the common steps (pp. 8-9).	To ensure that: • the patient is safe, comfortable and receiving the appropriate care; • results have been documented in the patient's records; • equipment is clean and in working order.

Evidence base: BTS (2008); Dougherty and Lister (2011); Smith and Roberts (2011); Smith (2012)

Measuring SpO$_2$

☑ **What is normal?**
Healthy adult 94%–98%
Adult with chronic chest problem e.g. COPD 88%–92%
Healthy infant (birth to 1 year) 95% –100%
Healthy child (over 1 year) 97%–99%

☑ **Before you start**
Remember the common steps for all clinical measurements (pp. 8–9).

Pulse oximetry only detects oxygen levels and not CO_2 levels

Other factors also need to be considered when measuring SpO$_2$ as this is not the only factor in detecting respiratory abnormalities. As you approach the patient observe for signs of hypoxia (severe lack of oxygen) by observing for central cyanosis (a blue/purple tint around the lips, earlobes, nose and upper chest). Does the patient appear to be breathing fast or slow, are they making any noises when breathing in or out and do they look as though the breathing is laboured?

☑ **Essential equipment**
Pulse oximeter

☑ **Care setting considerations**
SpO$_2$ can be measured in any care setting, as long as the equipment is available.

SpO$_2$ can be inaccurate if a patient has a saturation below 80%.

Dark skin pigmentation may reduce accuracy of the reading.

Step	Reason and patient-centred care considerations
1. Perform steps 1-8 of the common steps.	To prepare the patient and yourself to undertake the skill.
2. Select the probe size required for the chosen site: finger-tip, ear, toe, bridge of nose.	Pulse oximeter probes are available in different sizes and are designed for use with infants through to adults
3. Ensure that the site to be used is warm with a good circulation	The pulse oximeter requires a strong pulsatile signal to work. Poor tissue perfusion in conditions such as: hypovolaemia, hypotension, peripheral vascular disease, cardiac failure and some cardiac arrhythmias mean that the oximeter cannot pick up a signal or picks up a weak intermittent signal.
4. If the fingertips are being used remove any nail varnish and ensure fingers/nails are clean and dry.	Dark nail varnish can affect the translucency of the finger-tip reducing the accuracy of the reading.
5. Position the probe on the chosen site avoiding excess pressure.	Pulse oximeters can obstruct blood flow and cause pressure damage if positioned too tight or left in place for over 2 hours
6. Ensure all light emitting areas of the probe are in equal contact with the patient's skin.	If all light emitting areas of the probe are not in equal contact with the patient's skin the light may not be transmitted effectively. This may result in a falsely low reading.
7. Wait at least 7 seconds for the pulse oximeter to adjust and pick up a good waveform.	The pulse oximeter should record a waveform that corresponds to the beats you feel when taking the patient's radial pulse.
8. Perform steps 9-12 of the common steps	To ensure that the: • patient is safe, comfortable and receiving the appropriate care. • results have been documented in the patient's records • equipment is clean and in working order

Evidence base: BTS (2008); Dougherty and Lister (2011); Smith and Roberts (2011); Smith (2012)

☑ **What to watch out for and action to take**

If any abnormal recordings are observed this must be reported to a qualified nurse immediately and recorded in the patient's notes.

Abnormal SpO$_2$ values can sometimes be simple to improve by altering the patients position, ensuring they have adequate analgesia or increasing the amount of oxygen being administered to the patient. However, abnormal values must always be reported and acted upon as they can be an early sign of a patient's physiological deterioration.

☑ **Helpful Hints – Do I …?**

- Gloves and aprons must be worn if contact with blood/body fluids/excreta is anticipated or the patient is in isolation
- Hand hygiene must be performed before touching a patient, before clean/ aseptic procedures, after body fluid exposure/risk, after touching a patient and after touching a patient's surroundings
- Waste should be disposed of in a clinical waste bag if it is contaminated with blood/body fluids/excreta

Measuring a pulse rate (HR)

☑ **What is normal?**

- Adult range: 60–100 beats per minute (bpm)
- Child
  - Neonate (birth to 28 days) 100–180bpm
  - Infant (28 days to 1 year) 100–160bpm
  - Toddler (over 1 year to 3 years) 80–110bpm
  - Preschool (over 3 years to 5 years) 70–110bpm
  - School-aged children (over 5 years to 15 years) 65–110bpm
  - Adolescents (over 15 years to 17 years) 60–90bpm

☑ **Before you start**

Remember the common steps for all clinical measurements (pp. 8–9).

Most routine measurements of pulse rates are taken at the radial artery as this is easily accessible and does not compromise the patient's dignity.

For children under 1 year old the brachial artery or the apex are the best sites to palpate a pulse as their wrists tend not to be well defined, so finding a radial pulse is difficult.

In emergency life-threatening situations and to confirm cardiac arrest, the carotid and femoral pulses are often used.

☑ **Essential equipment**

Fob watch

Step				Reason and patient-centred care considerations
Perform steps 1-7 of the common steps (see pp. 8-9).				To prepare the patient and yourself to undertake the skill.
Radial pulse	**Brachial or apex pulse**	**Carotid pulse**	**Femoral pulse**	It is important to count the pulse rate for one minute as it is vital to assess whether the rhythm is regular and whether it has a good volume and quality. All of these factors can give you important information regarding a patient's cardiovascular status.
a. Ensure the patient's arm is resting on the chair arm, bed or couch. Place your second and third fingers over the inside of the wrist, in alignment with the thumb.	a. If you are unable to palpate a radial pulse in an adult the brachial artery is the next place to try as the artery is nearer to the heart and has a stronger pulsation. The apex or brachial palpation site is usually the best position to measure a pulse in a child. b. The brachial pulse can be found at the bend of the arm on the inside edge. This is diagonally across from the radial pulse.	a. Place your second and third fingers gently on the side of the neck approximately 5 cms down from the earlobe, slightly towards the throat.	a. Place your second and third fingers in the groin approximately 10 cms inwards from the hip.	
b. Once a rhythmic beat is felt count the number of times this occurs in 60 seconds (one minute).	c. The apex (or apical) pulse can be heard by placing a stethoscope at the fifth intercostal space (spaces between the ribs) on the chest, just left of the sternum. d. The same technique applies as taking a radial pulse.	b. Once a rhythmic beat is felt count the number of times this occurs in 60 seconds (one minute).	b. Once a rhythmic beat is felt count the number of times this occurs in 60 seconds (one minute).	
Perform steps 9-12 of the common steps (see pp. 8-9).				To ensure that: • the patient is safe, comfortable and receiving the appropriate care; • the results have been documented in the patient's records; • the equipment is clean and in working order.

Evidence base: Dougherty and Lister (2011); Smith and Roberts (2011); Smith (2012)

☑ Field-setting considerations

When taking an infant or child's pulse, the apex (apical) or brachial site is frequently used.

☑ Care-setting considerations

Pulse rates can be counted in any care setting, so long as the patient has not recently exercised or is not distressed or anxious.

☑ What to watch out for and action to take

If an abnormal pulse rate is counted or if you suspect an abnormality in the regularity or volume of the pulse rate, this must be reported to a qualified nurse immediately and recorded in the patient's notes.

Abnormal pulse rates can sometimes be simply improved through adequate analgesia and encouraging the patient to drink more fluid. However, abnormal values must always be reported and acted upon as they can be an early sign of a patient's physiological deterioration.

Automated blood pressure measurement (BP)

☑ What is normal?

Age	Systolic (mmHg)	Diastolic (mmHg)	Recorded as
Newborn	80	45	80/45 mmHg
10	105	70	105/70 mmHg
20	120	80	120/80 mmHg
40	125	85	125/85 mmHg
60	135	88	135/88 mmHg

A patient's normal BP is an individualized parameter and these values should be taken just as a guide.

☑ Before you start

Remember the common steps for all clinical measurements (pp. 8–9).

When recording a BP you need to consider which limb is the best to use. The site generally used is the upper 1/3rd of the arm as it is the most accessible; preferably the left arm due to its proximity to the aorta. However thighs and calves can be used with a correctly sized cuff. There are contraindications to using limbs when:

- **lymphoedema** is present
- the patient has had brachial artery surgery

- an **arteriovenous fistula** is present
- there is trauma to the limb

☑ **Essential equipment**

Automated Non Invasive Blood Pressure (NIBP) machine

☑ **Care setting considerations**

Automated machines can be used in any care setting.

☑ **What to watch out for and action to take**

Hypotension – A systolic blood pressure less than 90mmHg or a drop of 40mmHg from the patient's normal systolic blood pressure indicates Hypotension, which is a medical emergency, requiring rapid treatment and a search for the cause.

Hypertension – A systolic blood pressure greater than 140mmHg or a diastolic above 90mmHg reflects Hypertension and requires investigation (ALERT™ 2012).

☑ **Helpful Hints – Do I …?**
- Gloves and aprons must be worn if contact with blood/body fluids/excreta is anticipated or the patient is in isolation
- Hand hygiene must be performed before touching a patient, before clean/aseptic procedures, after body fluid exposure/risk, after touching a patient and after touching a patient's surroundings
- Waste should be disposed of in a clinical waste bag if it is contaminated with blood/body fluids/excreta

Step	Reason and patient-centred care considerations
1. Perform steps 1-8 of the common steps (pp. 8-9).	To prepare the patient and yourself to undertake the skill.
2. The patient should be in a comfortable position either sitting in a chair with legs uncrossed and feet flat on the floor or sitting/lying on a bed or couch with legs uncrossed. It is sometimes necessary to compare lying and standing blood pressures; in this case lying blood pressures should be taken first.	Inaccurate positioning of the patient, such as crossed legs can alter the BP reading.
3. Clothing on the limb where the BP is to be taken should be removed, if possible.	Clothing that restricts the blood flow in the limb where the BP is being taken can alter the reading.

Step	Reason and patient-centred care considerations
4. The arm should be resting on either the bed/couch, a chair arm, desk top or the patient's knee. Best practice is to place a pillow, blanket or item of clothing if available under the arm for support.	Accuracy of the BP reading is improved with a relaxed, well supported limb. The limb should be supported as near to the level of the heart as possible.
5. Cuffs are labelled with the size of the person that they are suitable for use with; such as large adult, standard adult, small adult, and child.	The wrong size cuff can reduce the accuracy of the measurement. Falsely high readings can occur with cuffs which are too small and falsely low readings can occur with cuffs which are too large. When the cuff is applied check that when wrapped around the arm the outside edges lie within the 2 large white lines, marked 'range'. If so, the cuff is the correct size and you will see that the cuff bladder (the part which inflates) is 80% of the arm circumference and 40% of its width. If this is not the case you need to apply a different size cuff.
6. Inside the cuff is a mark that should lie in line with the brachial artery. The lower edge of the cuff should be 2-3cms above the position where you put your fingers to palpate the brachial artery.	If the cuff is incorrectly positioned the accuracy of the measurement will be reduced.
7. Ask the patient to keep their arm still whilst the machine takes the reading.	Movement of the limb can reduce the accuracy of the measurement.
8. On most automated machines the start button is labelled NIBP (Non Invasive Blood Pressure) start. If the machine is having difficulty registering a BP or you want to stop the recording mid cycle there is a deflate NIBP button.	If a patient needs their blood pressure recorded frequently, for example every 15 minutes it is possible to set the automated machine to do this. However, remember to remove the cuff from the patient's limb at regular intervals as they can cause the skin to become hot, sweaty and cause marks or even sores on the skin.

Step	Reason and patient-centred care considerations
9. Perform steps 9-12 of the common steps (see pp. 8-9).	To ensure that the: • patient is safe, comfortable and receiving the appropriate care. • results have been documented in the patient's records. • equipment is clean and in working order.

Evidence base: BHS (2009); Dougherty and Lister (2011); Smith and Roberts (2011)

Manual blood pressure measurement (BP)

☑ **What is normal?**
Refer to Automated Blood Pressure Measurement (BP) (pp. 17–19).

☑ **Before you start**
Refer to Automated Blood Pressure Measurement (BP) (pp. 17–19).

☑ **Essential equipment**
Aneroid sphygmomanometer with stethoscope

☑ **Care-setting considerations**
Manual blood pressure measurements can be taken in any care setting.

☑ **What to watch out for and action to take**
Refer to Automated Blood Pressure Measurement (BP) (pp. 17–19).

Step	Reason and patient-centred care considerations
1. Perform steps 1-8 of the common steps (see pp. 8-9).	To prepare the patient and yourself to undertake the skill.
2. Perform steps 1-6 in automated blood pressure measurement (see pp. 17-19).	To ensure the patient is comfortable and correctly positioned, with a cuff of the appropriate size to enable accurate BP measurement.

Step	Reason and patient-centred care considerations
3. Position the sphygmomanometer no more than 1 metre away from the patient, upright, on a flat surface with the centre of the gauge at your eye level.	To ensure the measurement is as accurate as possible.
4. Check that your stethoscope is turned to the diaphragm side and working by tapping it with your finger.	To ensure your stethoscope is working and ready for use.
5. Palpate the patient's brachial artery, ensure that the valve is closed and then start pumping air into the cuff using the bulb. At the point when the pulse can no longer be felt provides a systolic estimation. The cuff should now be deflated.	By palpating the brachial pulse the correct position for the stethoscope can be located.
6. Deflate the cuff completely and wait 15–30 seconds.	This provides an approximate value of the systolic blood pressure. Allows venous congestion (dilated blood vessels due to the constriction caused by the cuff) to resolve.
7. Place the diaphragm of the stethoscope over the brachial artery where the pulse is palpable. Ensure the valve on the bulb attached to the cuff is closed firmly, but not so tightly that it cannot be deflated easily. Inflate the cuff again to 20–30mmHg above the predicted systolic blood pressure, as identified in step 6. Whilst observing the sphygmomanometer, slowly release the valve, at an approximate rate of 2-3 mmHg per pulsation, until the first thudding sounds are heard.	So you can listen for the sounds that will indicate the blood pressure. You will need to be able to manipulate the valve to inflate and deflate the cuff. Inflating the cuff will cause venous congestion. This is to compensate for an ausculatory gap and to ensure accuracy of measurement. These first thudding sounds are called the first Korotkoff sound and indicate the value for the systolic blood pressure. You need to note the pressure reading on the sphygmomanometer when you hear this sound.

Step	Reason and patient-centred care considerations
8. Continue to slowly release air from the valve, deflating the cuff. Listen carefully to the Korotkoff sounds until they disappear.	The disappearance of the Korotkoff sound is the value for the diastolic blood pressure - known as the Fifth Korotkoff sound. Again, you need to note the pressure reading on the sphygmomanometer when the Korotkoff sounds disappear.
9. Continue to slowly deflate the cuff another 20-30mmHg, until you are completely sure that all of the sounds have disappeared, then rapidly deflate the cuff.	To ensure your measurement is accurate. If the BP needs to be rechecked immediately, because the measurement is not what was expected or is too low or too high, wait for 1-2 minutes before proceeding.
10. Perform steps 9-12 of the common steps (see pp. 8-9).	To ensure that: • the patient is safe, comfortable and receiving the appropriate care; • results have been documented in the patient's records; • equipment is clean and in working order.

Evidence base: BHS (2009); Dougherty and Lister (2011); Smith and Roberts (2011)

Measuring capillary refill time (CRT)

☑ **What is normal?**
Normal range < 2 seconds (< means less than).

☑ **Before you start**
Remember the common steps for all clinical measurements.

☑ **Essential equipment**
None

☑ **Care setting considerations**
Can be measured in any care setting.

Peripheral CRT is usually measured by using the fingernail bed, but the toenail bed can also be used. If using the fingernail bed ensure the arm is at the level of the heart and if using the toenail bed ensure the leg is horizontal.

Central CRT can be assessed by pressing at the top of the sternum, using the same technique as fingernail bed or toenail bed.

☑ **What to watch out for and action to take**

Ask the patient if they have any problems with their peripheral circulation, for example Raynaud's disease, as this can prolong their CRT.

A prolonged CRT of greater than 2 seconds suggests poor peripheral perfusion. This may be normal if the patient is cold due to the ambient temperature, or if they are elderly or have a disease which reduces their peripheral circulation. A prolonged CRT in a limb that is warm, or if a patient is young and normally has good circulation requires further investigation.

Poor peripheral perfusion can be due to either a fall in BP and CO as the patient compensates by increasing their systemic vascular resistance (SVR) to ensure that blood flow to the vital organs of heart, brain, lungs, kidneys and liver is maintained for as long as possible.

☑ **Helpful Hints – Do I ...?**

Gloves and aprons must be worn if contact with blood/body fluids/excreta is anticipated or the patient is in isolation.

Hand hygiene must be performed before touching a patient, before clean/aseptic procedures, after body fluid exposure/risk, after touching a patient and after touching a patient's surroundings.

Waste should be disposed of in a clinical waste bag if it is contaminated with blood/body fluids/excreta.

Step	Reason and patient-centred care considerations
1. Perform steps 1-8 of the common steps (see pp. 8-9).	To prepare the patient and yourself to undertake the skill.
2. Assess the limb temperature as you raise the hand to the level of the heart or the leg horizontally. Do they feel cool or warm?	To determine whether it will be possible to use CRT to measure peripheral perfusion accurately. If the patient has cool limbs measuring central CRT will provide a more accurate reflection of their capillary refill time.
3. Apply sufficient pressure to cause blanching to the padded area of the fingertip or toe, or an area at the top of the sternum on the chest. Maintain this pressure for 5 seconds.	Using the padded areas of the finger is more reliable than using nails as they may be painted, acrylic, or it can be difficult to determine the change in colour.

Step	Reason and patient-centred care considerations
4. When the pressure is released assess how many seconds it takes for the skin to return to the colour of the surrounding skin.	This should occur in less than 2 seconds.
5. Perform steps 9-12 of the common steps (see pp. 8-9).	To ensure that the: • patient is safe, comfortable and receiving the appropriate care; • results have been documented in the patient's records.

Evidence base: ALS (2011); Smith (2012)

Measuring body temperature (T)

☑ **What is normal?**
Normal adult range 36.0–37.0° C.
Normal child range 36.6–37.7° C.

☑ **Before you start**
Remember the common steps for all clinical measurements (pp. 8–9).

☑ **Essential equipment**
The correct thermometer for the site you are using. A number of different types are available: oral, tympanic, temporal and axilla are the sites most often used.

☑ **Field-setting considerations**
You need to carefully consider which site is the most appropriate to use to measure your patient's temperature. For example, you would not use an oral thermometer if you were concerned that the patient might bite it, or if they had difficulty breathing through their nose. Tympanic thermometers are thought to be the most accurate and are used very frequently, but you would not use this site if a patient had wax or an infection in their ear canal or was younger than three months old.

Do not take a child's temperature immediately after they have had a bath or been wrapped in blankets, as this will not be an accurate recording.

☑ **Care-setting considerations**
Can be measured in any care setting.

Step	Reason and patient-centred care considerations		
1. Perform steps 1–8 of the common steps (pp. 8–9).	To prepare the patient and yourself to undertake the skill.		
Oral	**Tympanic**	**Temporal**	**Axilla**
2. Digital or disposable thermometers can be used to take oral temperatures. Attach the disposable probe cover and place the thermometer in the patient's mouth, positioned under their tongue, posteriorly into the sublingual pocket. Ask the patient to close their lips around the thermometer. Leave in this position for the specified amount of time. Read the temperature displayed. Dispose of the probe cover by pressing the RELEASE or EJECT button whilst holding	2. This is the most commonly used method of measuring temperature in adults as it is quick, minimally invasive and gives a rapid indication of a change in core temperature as the tympanic membrane is close to the hypothalamus. Remove the thermometer from the base unit. Check that the probe tip is clean and intact. Press the probe tip into the disposable probe cover without touching the cover. Gently pull the pinna (top of the ear) backwards so that the ear canal is	2. The temporal artery thermometer is held over the forehead to sense infrared emissions radiating from the skin. Hold in this position for the specified amount of time. Read the temperature displayed.	2. Digital or disposable thermometers can be used to take axilla temperatures. Place in the centre of the axilla and hold the arm close to the chest wall. Leave in this position for the specified amount of time. Read the temperature displayed. Dispose of the probe cover by pressing the RELEASE or EJECT button whilst holding over a

Reason and patient-centred care considerations (continued)

Oral

Factors affecting accuracy include the recent ingestion of food or fluid, a respiratory rate of greater than 18 bpm and smoking. Ensure the patient can breathe through their nose and is not at risk of biting the thermometer.

Tympanic

Avoid using this site if there has been a recent ear infection or there is wax in the ear canals as this can affect readings. Ask patients to remove any hearing aid if there is one in the ear to be used.

Use the same ear for readings as anatomical differences can account for a 1° difference.

If the ear canal is not straightened the reading will not be accurate

Step		Reason and patient-centred care considerations	
	Gently insert the thermometer into the ear canal until it is sealed.		**Temporal**
			Is quick to use but it has been shown to underestimate temperature.
	Press the scan button on the thermometer and wait for it to beep.		**Axilla**
	Gently remove the thermometer from the ear canal and read the temperature displayed.		Not as reliable as tympanic measurements for estimating core temperature as there are no main blood vessels around the axilla. Environmental temperature and perspiration can affect accuracy.
	Dispose of the probe cover by pressing the RELEASE or EJECT button whilst holding over a clinical waste bag.		
	Return to base unit.		
3.	Perform steps 9–12 of the common steps (see pp. 8–9).	To ensure that: • the patient is safe, comfortable and receiving the appropriate care; • the results have been documented in the patient's records; • the equipment is clean and in working order.	

Evidence base: Clancy and McVicar (2009); Dougherty and Lister (2011); Jevon (2010); McCallum and Higgins (2012); Smith and Roberts (2011)

Consider the environmental temperature's effect on the patient. It may feel warm to you, but the patient may be immobile and ill, so will need more clothing to keep them warm.

If the patient's temperature is raised, consider removing excess clothing.

☑ **What to watch out for and action to take**
Assessing your patient's temperature involves observation and feeling, as well as measurement. If the patient's temperature is elevated they may appear flushed and sweaty. When you are feeling their forehead or hands, they may feel hot to touch. Alternatively, if they are cold they may be shivering, wrapped in clothing or blankets and look pale, and their peripheries may feel cold to touch.

Blood glucose monitoring

☑ **What is normal**
4–7mmol/l

☑ **Before you start**
Remember the common steps for all clinical measurements.

Before taking the blood glucose monitoring device to the patient, the following blood glucose monitor checks need to be undertaken:

- Check test strips are in date and have not been exposed to air.
- The monitor and test strips have been calibrated together.
- If a new pack of strips are required, recalibrate the monitor.
- Complete any further quality control checks as per local guidelines.

☑ **Essential equipment**
Blood glucose monitor

Single use lance

Test strips

Sterile gauze

PPE

☑ **Care setting considerations**
Can be measured in any care setting.

When taking blood glucose measurements it is important to know when the patient last received food and any medication for blood glucose control, such as Insulin. Both of these factors can have an impact on the treatment given for abnormal blood glucose levels.

☑ What to watch out for and action to take

Abnormal glucose readings either high (hyperglycaemia) or low (hypoglycaemia) are a medical emergency and cause long term injury or death to the patient if not treated immediately. You must report abnormal findings to your mentor or a registered nurse immediately.

☑ Helpful Hints – Do I …?

Gloves and aprons must be worn if contact with blood/body fluids/excreta is anticipated or the patient is in isolation.

Hand hygiene must be performed before touching a patient, before clean/aseptic procedures, after body fluid exposure/risk, after touching a patient and after touching a patient's surroundings.

Waste should be disposed of in a clinical waste bag if it is contaminated with blood/body fluids/excreta.

Step	Reason and patient-centred care considerations
1. Perform steps 1-6 of the common steps (see pp. 8-9).	To prepare the patient and yourself to undertake the skill.
2. Select the finger to be lanced, involving the patient in making this decision as appropriate.	Placing the patient's hand below heart level will aid blood flow. Avoid index finger and thumb. Earlobes are a suitable alternative site for obtaining blood glucose samples. Never use toes for obtaining blood glucose samples. Do not use the same site repeatedly to reduce infection risk.
3. Using soap and water wash and dry the patient's hand/finger to be lanced.	Fingers need to be clean, as a contaminated sample will give an inaccurate result. The sample can be contaminated by: • Using alcohol gels and alcohol wipes to clean the finger. • Newspaper print, perfumes, hand creams, hairspray, hair gel. • The residue of food or drink on fingers.
4. Insert test strip following the manufacturer's guidelines into the strip port at the top of the meter. Wait for the flashing blood drop symbol to appear.	To prepare the glucometer.

Step	Reason and patient-centred care considerations
5. Prepare the single use lancing device by twisting and remove lancing device cap. Obtain the blood droplet from the patient by firmly pressing the lancing end against the chosen site. If using a finger, use the side. Remember to rotate the site. Depress the lancet fire clip. Dispose of used lancet in sharps bin.	The side of the finger is less painful and easier to obtain a hanging droplet of blood. Sites are rotated to avoid infection, to reduce pain from toughened skin. To avoid needle-stick injuries
6. Wait 5 seconds, then in continuous motion milk the blood flow. For example in a finger this would be from the palm of the hand down towards the tip of the finger. Never squeeze the finger or the area directly around the site.	This may result in inaccurate results from interstitial fluid in the sample.
7. Apply the blood to the strip. Ensure that the window on the test strip is entirely covered with blood. The blood glucose result will be displayed on screen in mmol/L.	The window on the test strip allows verification of a correctly dosed strip which needs to be covered to ensure accurate results.
8. Press firmly on puncture site with sterile gauze.	To stop bleeding.
9. Remove used test strip from meter.	
10. Perform steps 9-12 of the common steps (see pp. 8-9).	To ensure that the: • patient is safe, comfortable and receiving the appropriate care; • results have been documented in the patient's records; • equipment is clean and in working order.

Evidence base: Dougherty and Lister (2011)

PAIN MANAGEMENT

ANN KETTYLE

Undertaking a pain assessment

☑ **Before you start**

If the patient's notes are available, review them in order to gain as much information about the patient and their current situation as is possible.

Your assessment should not just focus on the pain itself but on whether the pain is new, recurring or persistent. It is helpful to ask the patient what medication they normally take for the pain, whether they have taken or done anything to alleviate the pain and, more importantly, whether it helped at all.

Gather the appropriate assessment tool and a pen.

☑ **Essential equipment**

Appropriate pain assessment tool

☑ **Field-specific considerations**

When caring for a patient with a learning disability it is important to know their level of understanding. You will need to allow time to explain what you are doing. It may be helpful to have the patient's family or carers present.

Patients who have mental health problems may not understand the relevance of what you are doing. Ensure you spend sufficient time explaining this. It may be helpful to have the patient's family or carers present.

Children, especially younger ones, may not understand what you are doing. It is often helpful to have parents or carers present to assist.

☑ **Care-setting considerations**

A pain assessment can be undertaken in any care setting.

Ensure that the setting is comfortable and private.

Always ensure that you use the most appropriate assessment tool available.

Comprehensive questions will provide you with an understanding of what pain is being experienced and indicate the most appropriate tool to be used on the next visit.

If you feel that the assessment was incomplete then you should arrange to return as soon as is convenient.

In an acute, hospital-based setting and once a full assessment has been completed, it is easier to provide medication or implement alternative strategies to help alleviate the pain; it is also easier to monitor the effects of the interventions as you see the patient more frequently. Outside the acute setting this becomes more difficult as you may only see the patient once a week or even less; however, visiting their home will give you the opportunity to observe how they cope with their pain, especially if it is chronic or persistent pain.

Reviewing a patient in their home setting affords you not only the opportunity to establish whether their normal medication is being taken as prescribed but also whether there is anything else that you can do for them, such as home adaptations.

☑ **What to watch out for and action to take**

Whilst undertaking a pain assessment you should also observe for non-verbal cues which may support the patient's answers or provide you with further information.

You should always ask to view the site of the pain and observe for signs of the following:

- Discolouration – any bruises, pale or reddened areas.
- Open areas or wounds and whether there is any exudate or bleeding.
- Swelling or inflammation around the site of the pain.
- The temperature of the skin around the site of the pain.
- If you are undertaking an initial pain assessment, you also need to consider whether the 'story' of the pain being described is alerting you to a safeguarding concern or whether it is identifying a possible life-threatening condition – for example, central chest pain may indicate serious heart damage.
- If you are undertaking a subsequent pain assessment make sure that you are able to review, compare and discuss any changes in the pain score provided by previous pain assessments with the patient and other healthcare professionals.

☑ **Helpful hints – Do I …?**

- Gloves and aprons must be worn if contact with blood/body fluids/excreta is anticipated or the patient is in isolation.
- Hand hygiene must be performed before touching a patient, before clean/ aseptic procedures, after body fluid exposure/risk, after touching a patient and after touching a patient's surroundings.
- Waste should be disposed of in a clinical waste bag if it is contaminated with blood/body fluids/excreta.

Step	Reason and patient-centred care considerations
1. The first step of any procedure is to introduce yourself to the patient, explain the procedure and gain their consent.	Fully informed consent may not always be possible if the patient is a child or has mental health problems or learning disabilities, but even in these circumstances, every effort should be made to explain the procedure in terms that the patient can understand. This is not only respectful of their individual human rights, but also helps to ensure that they will be more accepting of the treatment and that their anxieties are reduced.

For patients who are unable to provide consent because they are unconscious, advice should be sought from your mentor or another qualified nurse. |
| 2. Ask the patient whether it is acceptable to them for the assessment to be undertaken where they are. | If the patient wishes the assessment to be undertaken in a different area, find an appropriate location.

Ensure you maintain patient privacy, dignity and comfort at all times. |
| 3. Identify whether the patient is able to communicate with you or whether they want someone with them, such as an interpreter, family member or carer, to assist or support with the assessment. | Ensures that the patient is supported and their answers are communicated accurately in a timely manner. |
| 4. Prepare the environment, which includes making sure that the patient is:
• able to see you;
• as comfortable as possible (you may need to help them get into a comfortable position);
• in a position to have a private conversation.

Ensure that you position yourself at the patient's eye level with without risk to yourself. | To promote patient comfort and reduce anxiety.
Making sure that the conversation is taking place in a suitable environment will demonstrate respect for the patient and ensure that they feel able to communicate freely. |

Step	Reason and patient-centred care considerations
5. Throughout the assessment observe for non-verbal and visual signs of pain, such as sweating, grimacing, guarding, etc.	Enables you to identify whether the patient is 'holding back' or experiencing pain when they are unable to communicate with you. This is especially important in those with a learning disability or mental health need, where English is a second language and in the elderly, infirm or young children.
6. Talk to the patient in a gentle and unhurried manner. Do not talk too loudly but do make sure that you can be heard.	Effective communication is demonstrated and you are showing respect for the patient's feelings and experience.
7. Work through the assessment tool and listen to the patient's answers – if you are unclear ask them to elaborate or explain further.	Enables a comprehensive understanding of the patient's feelings and experience and the impact of their pain.
8. Document answers on a pain assessment tool and in 'patient' notes.	Accurate documentation allows for review of the efficacy of interventions and identification of further interventions.
9. If a patient identifies that they are in pain or you observe them to be in pain during the assessment, do not complete a full assessment but instead complete a primary assessment: • Where is the pain? • How long have they had it? • Have they had this pain before? • Have they taken anything for it? If so, did it work at all?	This primary assessment ensures that the patient is not left in pain for an unacceptable length of time. Do not delay obtaining appropriate pain relief – if the patient is in pain now then you need to act efficiently to ensure that they are treated as quickly as possible. Approach a doctor or nurse prescriber immediately to obtain directives for analgesia if you are in a hospital setting. If you are in the patient's own home ask them what they would like to take and whether you can get it for them, checking that the analgesia is being administered following the prescription.

Step	Reason and patient-centred care considerations
<ul><li>Are they allergic to anything?</li><li>Do they have any other conditions or take any other medication?</li><li>Other than medication, is there anything else they would like you to do to help relieve the pain?</li></ul> Administer medication and monitor effectiveness.	You can return later, when the patient is more comfortable, to complete the assessment. To ensure appropriate pain control.
10. On completion of the pain assessment, and if there are any previous assessments documented, compare and discuss with the patient the effect of any interventions previously provided or undertaken by themselves and identify the need for analgesia.	Pain assessments should be undertaken whenever the patient's vital signs are recorded or whenever the patient complains of pain. Comparison with previous pain assessments should be undertaken and the efficacy of any interventions reviewed to identify whether further strategies need to be implemented.
11. If any changes are noted report findings to your mentor, the doctor or senior nurse in charge and obtain a medication review as soon as possible.	This ensures that changes are addressed and that the patient's pain is controlled or that the patient is not on unnecessary medication.
12. Before leaving the patient ensure they are in a comfortable position, with drinks and call bells available as necessary.	Promotes patient comfort and ensures they are well nourished and hydrated.

Evidence base: NICE (2011a, 2013, 2014a); NMC (2010b); WHO (2009)

ASEPTIC TECHNIQUE AND SPECIMEN COLLECTION

ROSE GALLAGHER

Principles of asepsis

☑ Field-specific considerations

When caring for a patient with a learning disability it is important to be mindful of their level of understanding, so that consent and cooperation for the procedure can be gained. You will need to allow time to explain what you are doing and consider whether it will cause discomfort or pain.

Patients who have impaired mental capacity may not understand why you need to undertake an aseptic procedure. They may therefore withhold consent and you may need to refer to local policies on presumed or assumed consent, which will reflect requirements of the Mental Capacity Act 2005 and best interests.

As younger children may not understand what you wish to do, you may need to modify your approach – it may be helpful to have the parents or carers present to assist.

☑ Care-setting considerations

Aseptic technique can be undertaken in any care setting, although you may need to think carefully about how to best manage the patient's environment.

☑ What to watch out for and action to take

Whilst undertaking an aseptic procedure you should also assess:

- the general condition of the patient;
- their neurological condition – are they alert and responsive? Are they agitated?

- any signs or complaints of pain or discomfort;
- the patient's or relatives'/carers' views – for example saying that their condition is 'not quite right' or they 'don't feel well'.

The information gained from these observations is additional to any assessment you make relating to, for example, the wound you are dressing and will enable you to fully assess the patient's condition and institute appropriate treatment as necessary, escalating care needs to senior nurses and the medical team.

☑ **Helpful hints – Do I …?**
- Gloves and aprons must be worn if contact with blood/body fluids/ excreta is anticipated or the patient is in source isolation for IPC requirements.
- Hand hygiene must be performed before touching a patient, before clean/ aseptic procedures, after body fluid exposure/risk, after touching a patient and after touching a patient's immediate surroundings.
- Waste should be disposed of into the correct waste stream in line with a risk assessment.

Principle	Reason and patient-centred care considerations
Before you start	
1. Before commencing any care activity, introduce yourself to the patient, explain the procedure and gain their consent.	Fully informed consent may not always be possible if the patient is a child or has impaired mental capacity or learning disabilities, but even in these circumstances, every effort should be made to explain what you are going to do in terms that the patient can understand. This is not only respectful of their individual human rights, but also helps to ensure that they will be more accepting of the treatment and that their anxieties are reduced.
	For patients who are unable to provide consent because they are unconscious, refer to local policies.
2. Assess the procedure and determine its complexity before you start, collecting all equipment that may be needed (and an assistant if required).	To ensure you are fully prepared. This also avoids you having to leave the patient or interrupt the procedure.

Principle	Reason and patient-centred care considerations
3. Consider what is going on around you – do you really need to do an aseptic technique now (even if planned)?	To ensure that the environment is conducive to undertaking an aseptic technique. For example, there will be a negative environmental impact if bed-making or cleaning is being undertaken in close proximity to a large wound dressing being undertaken.
4. Ensure the patient is in a comfortable position where you can access the appropriate area. Ensure the patient has appropriate analgesia as required.	To promote patient comfort.
5. Clear sufficient space within the environment, for example around the bed space, chair or treatment area. Ensure the area is private.	Enables clear access for the patient and the nurse to work safely. Patients will feel exposed if others can see the care they are receiving. Maintain patient privacy, dignity and comfort as required.
6. Transport equipment to the patient appropriately (consider a dressing trolley if available and appropriate).	To ensure all equipment is to hand.
7. Perform hand hygiene and apply non-sterile gloves if required.	Wearing apron and gloves as part of personal protective equipment (PPE) is a standard infection prevention practice when dealing with body fluids or patients in isolation if they pose a risk of infection to others. Ensure your use of PPE is appropriate by considering the individual patient situation and the risk presented. Appropriate hand hygiene will assist in preventing and controlling infection.
Remove and dispose	
1. If present, remove any soiled dressings, 'contaminated' or 'dirty' items and place in appropriate waste bag according to risk assessment.	In preparation for dressing (etc.) change. Ensure soiled, contaminated or dirty items are disposed of appropriately.

Principle	Reason and patient-centred care considerations
2. Remove gloves and perform hand hygiene.	Appropriate hand hygiene will assist in preventing and controlling infection.
Create a 'sterile field'	
1. Open sterile pack and items, and create your 'sterile field' by placing only sterile items within this area.	Creating a sterile field avoids contamination through direct contact with non-sterile items. Remember your hands are not sterile!
2. Apply sterile or non-sterile gloves only if required.	A risk assessment will determine if sterile or non-sterile gloves are required.
3. Undertake procedure ensuring: • Only sterile items come into contact with the susceptible site. • Sterile and non-sterile items do not come into contact with each other.	In order to prevent and control infection.
To conclude	
1. After completing the care necessary ensure the patient is in a comfortable position, with drinks and call bells available as necessary.	Promotes patient comfort and ensures they are well nourished and hydrated.
2. Dispose of all waste and any single-use equipment, discard PPE (if used) and perform hand hygiene. Clean any equipment used as per the relevant policy every time it is used.	To prevent cross-infection and maintain equipment in working condition.
3. Document the care provided in the patient's notes.	Maintains patient safety and accurate records.
4. If any abnormal findings are observed, report to mentor or a registered nurse immediately.	It is vital to report abnormal findings to a registered nurse immediately so they can ensure care is escalated. Failure to do so can result in the patient's condition deteriorating, and potentially preventable adverse outcomes.

Evidence base: Loveday et al. (2013); NICE (2012a); WHO (2009)

Common steps for the collection of all types of specimen

☑ **Essential equipment – depends upon the specimen but is likely to include one or more of the following**
Specimen container, specimen bag and laboratory form
Swabs as appropriate

☑ **Field-specific considerations**
When collecting a specimen from a patient with a learning disability it is important to know their level of understanding so that consent and cooperation can be gained. You will need to allow time to explain what you are doing, why you are doing it and whether it will cause discomfort or pain.

Patients who have impaired mental capacity may not understand why you need to collect a specimen. They may therefore withhold consent and you may need to refer to local policies on presumed or assumed consent, which will reflect requirements of the Mental Capacity Act 2005 and best interests.

Younger children may not understand why you need to collect a specimen. You will need to adopt an appropriate approach. It may be helpful to have the parents or carers present to assist.

☑ **Care-setting considerations**
Specimens can be collected in all care settings.

☑ **Key points to remember**
- There is a clear clinical need for the specimen.
- Explain rationale to patient and gain consent.
- Specimen must be obtained without contamination.
- Specimen must be stored appropriately or transferred to laboratory as soon as possible.
- Check result and act on it accordingly.

☑ **Helpful hints – Do I …?**
- Gloves and aprons must be worn if contact with blood/body fluids/excreta is anticipated or the patient is in isolation.
- Hand hygiene must be performed before touching a patient, before clean/aseptic procedures, after body fluid exposure/risk, after touching a patient and after touching a patient's surroundings.
- Waste should be disposed of in a waste bag if it is contaminated with blood/body fluids/excreta in line with risk assessment for waste.

Step	Reason and patient-centred care considerations
1. The first step of any procedure is to introduce yourself to the patient, explain the procedure and gain their consent.	Fully informed consent may not always be possible if the patient is a child or has impaired mental capacity or learning disabilities, but even in these circumstances, every effort should be made to explain the procedure in terms that the patient can understand. This is not only respectful of their individual human rights, but also helps to ensure that they will be more accepting of the treatment and that their anxieties are reduced.

For patients who are unable to provide consent because they are unconscious, local policies should be referred to. |
| 2. Ensure that it is an appropriate time to collect the specimen. | The quality of the specimen can be affected by the time of collection and length of time before it reaches the laboratory. To ensure the specimen is of the best quality, ensure that it will reach the laboratory quickly once it has been collected and that it is the best time of day to collect the specimen. For example, it is best to collect a urine sample from the first voided urine in the morning for mycobacterial culture as this will contain the highest concentration of bacteria present. |
| 3. Gather the equipment required to collect the specimen; ensure this is clean and in working order. | Reduces the chance of inaccurate results.

All lids, containers and specimen bags should be checked to ensure there are no leaks or breaches which could result in spillage during transportation.

Containers used for the collection and transport of specimens should be CE-marked as this confirms that the container complies with essential requirements – only approved containers should contain specimens for laboratory analysis.

This reduces the chance of infection, and helps maintain the quality of the specimen. |

Step	Reason and patient-centred care considerations
4. Clear sufficient space within the environment where the specimen is to be collected, for example around the bed space or chair.	Enables clear access for the patient and the nurse to safely use the equipment required.
5. Standard IPC precautions should be used whenever there is a need to collect specimens.	Wearing an apron and gloves as part of personal protective equipment (PPE) is a standard infection-control procedure when dealing with body fluids or patients in isolation. Ensure your use of PPE such as gloves and disposable aprons is appropriate by considering the individual patient's situation and the risk presented.
6. Patients need to be in a private, comfortable and appropriate position and surroundings.	Maintain patient privacy, dignity and comfort as required. To promote patient comfort and reduce anxiety.
7. Complete the appropriate laboratory forms.	The information provided on specimen or laboratory forms is very important. Incorrectly spelled or wrong patient names and identifying information could result in the wrong result being placed in a patient's notes. Alternatively, poorly completed forms could result in specimens being rejected by the laboratory, with significant implications for the patient.

Step	Reason and patient-centred care considerations
	Some organizations use electronically generated specimen request forms and specimen labels to support laboratory tests. Always check local policies for more information.
The laboratory request form must include the following information: • Patient surname and forename (care should be taken to avoid use of nicknames). • Date of birth. • Gender. • NHS or hospital number – refer to local policies regarding patient unique identifiers and their use. • Location of where specimen obtained (if relevant). • Requesting clinician or consultant in charge. • Sample date and time. • Name or initial of the person taking the specimen. • Clinical information relevant to the specimen – this helps laboratory staff to interpret the clinical significance of specimen results. Examples include symptoms, possible or confirmed diagnosis, any current treatment (e.g. antibiotics) and other pertinent history such as foreign travel.	
8. Double-check to ensure the patient is correctly identified – ask the patient (where possible) to state their full name and date of birth. Use patient identifiers (e.g. wristbands) where possible to confirm.	Prevents you from taking a specimen from the wrong patient. Never ask 'are you ...?' Always ask the patient to state their name and date of birth. Some patients may not wear wristbands, e.g. neonates, those living in care homes or those with amputated limbs – check your local policies for alternatives to wristbands.

Step	Reason and patient-centred care considerations
9. Ensure specimen is collected in line with local policy.	Using an aseptic technique reduces the risk of contaminating the specimen.
10. Specimens for microbiological investigation should ideally be taken before antibiotic therapy is commenced.	If the patient is already on antibiotics before a specimen is taken, this may have a significant impact on identification of the causative organism (bacteria). The laboratory must be informed on the laboratory form of all therapy the patient is receiving or has recently received.
11. Specimens for viral investigation can require special transport media.	Viruses are generally quite fragile and die easily. Examples include chickenpox (varicella), chlamydia, influenza, norovirus. Where specimens are taken directly from lesions, such as vesicles of herpes or chickenpox, then the swab must be placed inside special viral transport media to preserve any viral particles during transport to the laboratory. Viral transport media may require refrigeration and will have an expiry date. Refer to local policies for more information.
12. Label container and seal in the specimen bag along with the laboratory request form, in line with local policy.	Ensures the specimen and laboratory form are retained together and avoids loss of either during transport.

Step	Reason and patient-centred care considerations
13. Specimens should be transported to the laboratory and processed as soon as possible.	Once a specimen is obtained, any micro-organisms present have been removed from their 'natural' habitat; therefore in order to preserve micro-organisms, transport to the laboratory should take place as soon as possible. If there is a delay in transportation, some specimens may be refrigerated in a designated refrigerator (do not put in a food fridge) until collection. This is preferable to leaving them at room temperature, which could interfere with the laboratory interpretation of results.

For some specimens, delays of over 48 hours are considered unsatisfactory as the specimen will have deteriorated. Check local policy for further guidelines. |
14. After collecting the specimen ensure the patient is in a comfortable position, with drinks and call bells available as necessary.	Promotes patient comfort and ensures they are well nourished and hydrated.
15. Discard PPE, any single-use equipment and other used materials as per policy. Clean any equipment used as per the relevant policy and perform hand hygiene.	To prevent cross-infection and maintain equipment in working condition.
16. Document the specimen collection in the patient's notes.	Maintains patient safety and accurate records.

Evidence base: WHO (2009)

Taking a wound swab

Wounds include surgical and traumatic wounds, burns, ulcers, folliculitis and invasive device insertion sites such as an intravenous cannula or wound drain.

Indications for taking the specimen
Wound infection, cellulitis (in the presence of a break in the skin) and/or the presence of pus:

The presence of bacteria in a wound without signs and symptoms of infection reflects colonization only, and is common in chronic wounds (such as leg ulcers in community settings).

Step	Reason and patient-centred care considerations
1. Perform steps 1-8 of the common steps (see pp. 39-43).	To prepare the patient and yourself to undertake the task.
2. Dip swab in transport media (if present with swab) or moisten with sterile saline.	To preserve any bacteria present during transportation to the laboratory. Moisten swab to avoid dessication of any bacteria present.
3. If pus is present collect pus (via aspiration) or use a moistened swab.	To preserve any bacteria present during transportation to the laboratory.
4. Take swab from the part of the wound exhibiting symptoms of infection.	This area will produce the best results.
5. Using an aseptic technique perform a 'zig-zag' motion whilst gently rotating the swab between the fingers.	To ensure good contact by the swab with the wound.
6. Place the wound swab immediately back into the container.	To prevent contamination.

Step	Reason and patient-centred care considerations
7. Perform steps 10-16 of the common steps (see pp. 39-43).	To ensure that: • the patient is safe and comfortable. • the specimen has been correctly collected and documented in the patient's records. • the equipment is clean and in working order.

Evidence base: PHE (2014a)

Collecting a faeces specimen

Indications for taking the specimen

Gastro-intestinal infections (bacterial, viral or parasitic) e.g. food poisoning (Salmonella, Campylobacter, Giardia), C. *difficile*, Norovirus, Shigella, tapeworm.

Ensure the patient actually has diarrhoea in line with local definitions, check with patient if possible and refer to stool chart.

If the patient has previously been diagnosed with C. *difficile* infection check with your local infection prevention team and policies for guidance on whether further specimens are required.

Step	Reason and patient-centred care considerations
1. Perform steps 1-8 of the common steps.	To prepare the patient and yourself to undertake the skill.
2. Negotiate with the patient for them to defecate into a commode or bedpan.	To enable a sample to be collected. Support the patient to avoid urinating at the same time. To maintain accurate documentation remember to record specimen collection and bowel motion on stool chart.

Step	Reason and patient-centred care considerations
3. Place sample in specimen container carefully avoiding contamination of the outside of the pot.	A maximum of 10g of faeces is suitable for investigation. **Do not overfill the container** due to the risk of explosion on opening in the laboratory – natural gases are produced by faecal bacteria so if the specimen is stored in warm conditions a buildup of gas can occur resulting in explosion on opening (with potentially unpleasant results!).
4. Ensure faeces specimens are transported to the laboratory as soon as possible.	Some important organisms e.g. Shigella cysts do not survive well if specimens are delayed for any length of time.
5. Perform steps 10-16 of the common steps.	To ensure that the: • patient is safe and comfortable. • specimen has been correctly collected and documented in the patient's records. • equipment is clean and in working order.

Evidence base: PHE (2014b)

Collecting a urine specimen

A urine sample includes mid-stream (MSU), clean catch (CCU) and catheter specimen of urine (CSU). Early morning urine (EMU) is required for some tests.

Patients may require support from nursing staff to collect an MSU if they have mobility problems, are elderly or have learning disabilities. Some patients also find the thought of collecting specimens distasteful or undignified and may require support from staff with this. Commercial kits are now available that incorporate a funnel to help patients 'aim' urine into the container and avoid contamination of the outside of the container.

Indications for taking the specimen
Suspected urinary tract infection, other investigation e.g. legionella antigen test.

EMU for renal tuberculosis or hormonal investigations.

Step			considerations
1. Perform steps 1-8 of the common steps (see pp. 39-43).			To prepare the patient and yourself to undertake the skill.
Mid-stream specimen (MSU)	**Clean catch specimen (CCU)**	**Catheter specimen (CSU)**	**MSU and CCU**
2. Advise patient on how to collect the specimen.		2. Samples may be obtained from a urethral or supra pubic catheter or as a result of intermittent self-catheterization.	Advice relating to how to collect the specimen will differ according to whether the patient is male or female because of anatomical differences in the urogenital area.
3. The sample should be collected by advising the patient not to urinate immediately into the container but to discard the first few mls of urine. The first few mls of urine may become contaminated during voiding which could affect the sample quality.	3. All urine is voided into a sterile container and then a portion of this is decanted into a sterile urine specimen container. The laboratory request form must be clear that the urine is a CCU and not an MSU to support laboratory interpretation of results.	3. The sample should be removed using a syringe from the dedicated port on the catheter. The specimen should never be taken from the tap of the catheter bag. The sampling port should be cleaned with an alcohol wipe if physically clean (if soiled it may be necessary to clean first with detergent and water or detergent wipe).	For both male and female patients peri-urethral cleaning is recommended, water is sufficient for this. Separate swabs should be used for each wiping motion and in females the wiping motion should be from front to back to avoid contamination from the anal region. A CCU is not as good quality as an MSU but is a reasonable alternative where an MSU cannot be obtained.

Step	Reason and patient-centred care considerations
	CSU Aseptic technique is used to reduce the infection risk. Historically CSUs were collected using a needle and syringe to access urine via a self-sealing sampling sleeve. This practice is no longer acceptable due to the risk of needle-stick injury.
4. As necessary place sample in specimen container carefully avoiding contamination of the outside of the pot.	10ml of urine is sufficient for microbiological investigations.
5. Perform steps 10-16 of the common steps.	To ensure that the: • patient is safe and comfortable. • specimen has been correctly collected and documented in the patients records. • equipment is clean and in working order.

Evidence base: PHE (2014c); Sharp Instruments in Healthcare Regulations (2013)

Collecting a sputum sample

Indications for taking the specimen

Upper and lower respiratory tract infections, including pneumonia:

Micro-organisms normally present in the upper respiratory tract can contaminate the usually sterile lower respiratory tract and cause infection.

Green sputum does not necessarily mean the patient has an infection!

Step	Reason and patient-centred care considerations
1. Perform steps 1-8 of the common steps (see pp. 39-43).	To prepare the patient and yourself to undertake the skill.
2. The patient is required to expectorate in order to produce a specimen of sputum - saliva is not suitable.	Patients who have difficulty coughing or expectorating may need a physiotherapist to help them produce a sample.
3. As necessary, place sample in specimen container, carefully avoiding contamination of the outside of the pot.	A minimum of 1 ml of sputum is required.
4. Samples should be sent to the laboratory as soon as possible (sputum may be refrigerated for up to 2-3 hours).	Some bacteria die easily and overgrowth of other bacteria occurs quickly at room temperature, which will produce false results.
5. Perform steps 10-16 of the common steps (see pp. 39-43).	To ensure that: • the patient is safe and comfortable. • the specimen has been correctly collected and documented in the patient's records. • the equipment is clean and in working order.

Evidence base: PHE (2014e)

Taking a nasal swab

Indications for taking the specimen
To detect clinically important bacteria in the nose, for example to determine if the patient is colonized with a bacteria such as meticillin-resistant *Staphylococcus aureus* (MRSA) or meticillin-sensitive *Staphylococcus aureus* (MSSA).

Step	Reason and patient-centred care considerations
1. Perform steps 1-8 of the common steps (see pp. 39-43).	To prepare the patient and yourself to undertake the skill.
2. Dip swab in transport media (if present with swab) or moisten with sterile saline. One swab can be used to swab both nostrils.	To preserve any bacteria present during transportation to the laboratory. Moisten swab to avoid dessication of any bacteria present.
3. Swabs must be taken from the anterior nares of the nose. The swab should be inserted just inside the nostrils and then directed gently upwards back towards the tip of the nose and rotated to ensure gentle contact with the mucosal surface.	The anterior nares are the external part of the nostrils.
4. Perform steps 10-16 of the common steps (see pp. 39-43).	To ensure that: • the patient is safe and comfortable. • the specimen has been correctly collected and documented in the patient's records. • the equipment is clean and in working order.

Evidence base: Dougherty and Lister (2011); PHE (2015)

Taking a throat swab

Indications for taking the specimen

To detect a throat infection or carriage of clinically important bacteria, such as MRSA, or occasionally for screening in outbreak or contact situations with, for example, Group A Streptococci, *N. meningitides*.

Step	Reason and patient-centred care considerations
1. Perform steps 1-8 of the common steps (see pp. 39-43).	To prepare the patient and yourself to undertake the procedure.
2. Depress the tongue to expose the fauces of the tonsils and gently and quickly rub the swab over the affected or inflamed area.	Ensure you have good lighting present to enable you to see into the throat. The fauces or 'pillars of fauces' are two membranous folds which enclose the tonsils. Rubbing the swab over the affected area may make the patient gag, obstructing the view of the tonsils. Avoid contact between the swab and other parts of the mouth (tongue and teeth) as this will contaminate the swab.
3. Perform steps 10-16 of the common steps (see pp. 39-43).	To ensure that: • the patient is safe and comfortable. • the specimen has been correctly collected and documented in the patient's records. • the equipment is clean and in working order.

Evidence base: PHE (2014d)

SKIN INTEGRITY

IRENE ANDERSON AND CATHERINE DELVES-YATES

Principles of caring for a patient with a wound

☑ **Essential equipment**

This will depend upon patient need and the type of care being undertaken but is likely to include some of the following: analgesia, dressings and equipment to clean the wound aseptically.

Always ensure any equipment is clean and in working order before you use it.

☑ **Field-specific considerations**

When caring for a patient with a learning disability it is important to know their level of understanding so that consent for and cooperation with the wound-related care can be gained. You will need to allow time to explain what you are doing and whether your actions will cause discomfort or pain.

Patients who have mental health problems may not understand the relevance of what you are doing. Ensure you spend sufficient time explaining this. It may be helpful to have the patient's family or carers present.

Younger children may not understand why you need to perform wound-related care; this will determine your approach to undertaking the procedure. It is usually helpful to have the parents or carers present to assist.

☑ **Care-setting considerations**

Wound-related care can be performed in both hospital and community care settings as long as the equipment required is available.

☑ **What to watch out for and action to take**

Whilst delivering wound-related care you should also use your observations to assess the patient's condition. For example, it is possible to assess:

- the colour of the skin, lips and nail beds for signs of cyanosis;
- the patient's positioning and how they are moving;
- their neurological condition – are they alert and responsive?;
- any signs or complaints of pain or discomfort;
- the patient's or relatives' views – for example saying that their condition is 'not quite right' or they 'don't feel well'.

The information gained from these observations is additional to the wound care procedure but enables you to fully assess the patient's condition and institute appropriate treatment as necessary, escalating any concerns to senior nurses and the medical team.

☑ **Helpful hints – Do I …?**
- Gloves and aprons must be worn if contact with blood/body fluids/excreta is anticipated or the patient is in isolation.
- Hand hygiene must be performed before touching a patient, before clean/aseptic procedures, after body fluid exposure/risk, after touching a patient and after touching a patient's surroundings.
- Waste should be disposed of in a clinical waste bag if it is contaminated with blood/body fluids/excreta.

Equipment must be cleaned as identified by the relevant policy every time it is used.

Steps	Reason and patient-centred care considerations
1. The first step of any procedure is to introduce yourself to the patient, explain the procedure and gain their consent.	Fully informed consent may not always be possible if the patient is a child or has mental health problems or learning disabilities, but even in these circumstances, every effort should be made to explain the procedure in terms that the patient can understand. This is not only respectful of their individual human rights, but also helps to ensure that they will be more accepting of the treatment and that their anxieties are reduced. For patients who are unable to provide consent because they are unconscious, advice should be sought from your mentor or another qualified nurse.
2. Gather any equipment required. Ensure this is clean as appropriate and in working order.	Reduces the chance of infection and maintains patient and nurse safety.
3. Clear sufficient space within the environment, for example around the bed space or chair.	Enables clear access for the patient and the nurse to safely use the equipment required.

Steps	Reason and patient-centred care considerations
4. Wash your hands with soap and water. Apron and gloves should only be worn if appropriate.	Wearing an apron and gloves as part of personal protective equipment (PPE) is a standard infection-control procedure when dealing with body fluids or patients in isolation. Ensure your use of PPE such as gloves and disposable aprons is appropriate by considering the individual patient situation and the risk presented.
5. Close the curtains or take other appropriate measures to maintain the patient's privacy.	Maintain patient privacy, dignity and comfort as required.
6. Identify the healing stage of the wound (using the information provided in Appendix 4, p. 191-192).	Identifying the healing stage of the wound will enable you to provide the most effective care. Ensure the care you deliver focuses upon the priorities identified.
Stage 1: Haemostasis	In order for the wound healing process to start, the bleeding has to stop. To do this, elevate the limb affected (where possible) and apply localized pressure to start the clotting process. The patient may be shocked and in pain so it is important they are reassured, basic first aid principles are applied and appropriate help is sought. If the patient is in pain, this must also be treated as a priority.
Stage 2: Inflammation	Slough and necrotic tissue needs to be removed from the wound (debridement) as it can delay healing by causing a barrier to cell movement, and can potentially harbour infection. Pain relief, immobilization and protection of the wound site are necessary. The use of antiseptics should be avoided unless there is a risk of infection, because the presence of inflammation is normal at this stage of the wound healing process. Wounds which have occurred in 'dirty' conditions (e.g. trauma) may need immediate antimicrobial therapy, but this should not be a matter of routine.
	Patient-related factors may reduce the inflammatory response needed for optimum wound healing. For example, patients on long-term steroid therapy or with poorly controlled diabetes, cardiovascular disease or an inflammatory condition such as rheumatoid arthritis will not experience a full inflammatory response. This will result in a reduced inflammation phase of healing, so the wound care provided must take all of these factors into account.

Steps	Reason and patient-centred care considerations
Stage 3: Proliferation	At this stage the wound requires warmth, moisture and protection from damage.
	The patient will require regular pain assessment and management, as well as reassurance about the progress of the wound.
	Pale granulation tissue (rather than healthy red) may indicate a lack of tissue oxygen (ischaemia), which is possible if the patient has a cardiac condition. Granulation tissue that is dark red and/or bleeding spontaneously may indicate infection.
	If granulation is allowed to dry out, due to prolonged exposure of the wound to air or an inappropriate dressing, then the cell activity may slow down and healing will be delayed. In very exceptional circumstances a dry wound may be preferred (e.g. necrotic fingers or toes in a patient with diabetes), but normally the wound should be moist and warm.
	Children or patients with cognitive impairment may need extra support to protect delicate granulation tissue from harm through scratching or other damage.
Stage 4: Maturation	The patient needs to be educated that healing is still continuing although signs may not be obvious.
	Although the wound has repaired, there will be scar tissue. The patient, family or carers may be anxious about the appearance of the scar tissue, which may be red and standing proud of the surrounding skin. Normally, over time, this will become paler and flatter. However, in some cases there may be abnormal scarring, where the tissue remains red and raised (hypertrophic). A less common type of scarring is keloid, where scar tissue remains prominent and may spread beyond the boundaries of the original wound. Scarred areas should be protected from injury, sun damage and excessive dryness as part of a good skin care regime, and scratching should be particularly avoided as this will damage newly healed skin.
7. After performing wound-related care ensure the patient is in a comfortable position, with drinks and call bells available as necessary.	Promotes patient comfort and ensures they are well nourished and hydrated.
8. Discard PPE, any single-use equipment and other used materials as per policy.	To prevent cross-infection and maintain equipment in working condition.

Steps	Reason and patient-centred care considerations
Clean any equipment used as per the relevant policy every time it is used and perform hand hygiene.	
9. Document the care provided, and if necessary any findings, on the patient's observation chart and/ or in the patient's notes.	Maintains patient safety and accurate records.
10. If any abnormalities are observed, escalate to senior nursing staff/ mentor immediately.	It is vital to report abnormal findings to a registered nurse immediately so they can ensure care is escalated. Failure to do so can result in the patient's condition deteriorating, potentially leading to death.

Evidence base: Dougherty and Lister (2011); Trott (2005); WHO (2009)

Pressure related injuries - quick reference guide

☑ Definition
A pressure related injury is 'localized injury to the skin and/or underlying tissue usually over a bony prominence, as a result of pressure, or pressure in combination with shear' (EPUAP 2014).

Helpful hint – Remember that the pressure injury may not always be over a bony prominence.

☑ Cause
Either from pressure over bony areas or from an external source – such as a splint, collar, frame, plaster cast or occasionally friction. Pressure of any type leads to a loss of skin integrity, discolouration, reduced perfusion, skin break down, **ischaemia** and ulceration.

☑ Grading
1. Non-blanchable erythema.

   The ulcer appears as a red area (on lightly pigmented skin) or a red, blue or purple hue (on darker skin tones),which does not resolve 30 minutes after the pressure has been removed. Skin is intact.

2. Partial thickness.

    Skin is broken but the lesion is superficial with no measureable depth.

3. Full thickness skin loss.

    A break through the dermis of the skin and possibly including damage or necrosis of subcutaneous tissue.

4. Full thickness tissue loss.

    A break through all of the skin layers extending into muscle, tendon and bone.

    An additional category of 'unstageable' is used where the actual depth of the ulcer is not visible due to thick slough (EPUAP 2014).

Helpful hint – Remember that pressure ulcers of all stages are painful. Ensure you assess a patient's pain frequently with a pain scale that is appropriate for their cognitive level. Dressing changes can be very painful, so always ensure that analgesia has been considered if the patient finds the dressing change uncomfortable or painful, and constantly assess the pain the patient is experiencing.

☑ Prevention
- Assessment of patient comfort.
- Moving and handling assessment and care planning.
- Completion of tissue viability score within 6 hours of admission.
- Regular repositioning of a patient – at least 2 hourly.
- Careful moving and handling techniques – to prevent shearing of skin.
- Assessment and timely use of pressure relieving aids, such as special mattresses and cushions to help redistribute pressure.
- Ensure bed linen is dry and free from creases – to reduce risk of skin damage.
- Effective hygiene – to keep skin clean and dry.
- Ensure adequate nutrition and hydration – to promote healthy tissues.

☑ Risk Assessment
NICE guidelines (2014b) state that patients should have a pressure ulcer risk assessment within six hours of admission and regularly thereafter. There are a wide range of risk assessment tools. The most well-known is Waterlow (2005) although there are many others such as Braden (1997), and Norton (Schoonhoven et al., 2002). There are also tools specifically for neonates and children (Willock et al., 2009). Whilst risk assessment tools are means of achieving a structured approach to assessing a patient, clinical judgement is also vital to ensure that the correct preventative strategies are put in place.

☑ **Evidence base:** Braden (1997); EPUAP (2014); NICE (2014b); Piper et al. (2009); Schoonhoven et al. (2002); Waterlow (2005); Willock et al. (2009)

SAFER HANDLING OF PEOPLE

DIANNE STEELE

Efficient movement principles

☑ **Care-setting considerations**

For your health and safety you must always apply efficient movement principles in all care settings.

Steps	Reason and patient-centred care considerations
1. Ensure you establish a stable base. The body's balance is enhanced when the feet are placed further apart, but to a degree still remains unstable if a force is applied laterally.	To ensure we are in the correct position to assist a patient to move. We rarely stand with our feet together or touching. If we do adopt this position it is only for a short period. The body is not designed to take this stance because it needs to be alert and ready to move.
For almost all manual handling manoeuvres one foot should be placed forwards and the other behind and with the leg bent at the knee, as this provides a stable base. The stride stand is the start of movement. It allows the body to move by bending the knee, allowing the worker to flex at the hips whilst maintaining the 'S' shape of the spine.	This maintains a natural relaxed posture. The forward movement will require the back extensor and abdominal muscles to engage, as well as the gluteus medius, quadriceps and hamstring muscles controlling the hips, legs and knees. These all assist in stability and maintain the centre of gravity.

Steps	Reason and patient-centred care considerations
	Always remember feet control a stable base and allow movement, so ensure you consider how you can best achieve this when working around beds, chairs, baths, low surfaces and confined working spaces, especially those in the community setting.
2. Knees and hips. These must be slightly flexed.	To assist in free movement and enable the individual to be relaxed.
3. Spinal column. The spine should not be in tension but should maintain the natural 'S' shape, with little flexion, lateral bending or trunk torsion.	Adopting a 'C' shape in the spine suggests increased hip and lumbar flexion, which will result in you adopting a stooping posture – thoracic kyphosis.
4. Head alignment. The position of the head should be raised but not extended. Placing the chin in a neutral position encourages the thoracic and lumbar regions to adopt their natural position.	Ensure you avoid extension, flexion or twisting of the neck.
5. Arms. The position of the arms is important for maintaining balance because they act as levers. You should keep your arms and elbows near to your body, flexed and aligned to the hips. Your hand placement must be non-invasive and must neither grip nor cause discomfort to the patient.	Arms and elbows rarely work independently, but rely on foot, hip and back movement. The arms add the refinement of movement because the position of the hands and wrists acts as the connecting force to the load.
6. Breath control. When we apply a force to move a person or object, we momentarily hold our breath.	As we breathe in, the diaphragm moves downwards, increasing the space available to the expanding lungs. At the same time the abdominal muscles contract, increasing the intra-abdominal pressure. This pressure acts as a splint for our front and we

Steps	Reason and patient-centred care considerations
	are supported at the back by the muscles of the spine. So, momentary breath-holding is beneficial and becomes part of a safer handling manoeuvre.
	Just don't forget to start breathing again.

Evidence base: HSE (2000, 2004); Marieb (2013); Polak (2011); Smith (2011); NMC (2015)

A safe way of working when moving a patient

☑ **Before you start**
Ensure you perform a thorough risk assessment.

☑ **Essential equipment**
This will depend upon patient need and type of move being undertaken but is likely to include some of the following: hoist, sling, stand and turn aids, transfer aids, glide sheets. Always ensure any equipment is clean and in working order before you use it. Refer to local policy and manufacturers' instructions.

☑ **Field-specific considerations**
When caring for a patient with a learning disability it is important to know their level of understanding so that consent for and cooperation with the move can be gained. You will need to allow time to explain what you are doing and whether your actions will cause discomfort or pain.

Patients who have mental health illness may not understand the relevance of what you are doing. Ensure you spend sufficient time explaining this. It may be helpful to have the patient's family or carers present.

Younger children may not understand why you need to move them; this will determine your approach to undertaking the move. It is usually helpful to have the parents or carers present to assist.

☑ **Care-setting considerations**
With sufficient care and planning, safer moving and handling can be performed in both hospital and community care settings as long as the equipment required is available.

☑ **What to watch out for and action to take**

Whilst moving a patient you should also use your observation skills to assess the patient's condition. For example, when moving a patient it is possible to assess:

- the colour of the skin, lips and nail beds for signs of cyanosis;
- their previous position;
- their neurological condition – are they alert and responsive?
- any signs or complaints of pain or discomfort;
- the patient's or relatives' views – for example, saying that their condition is 'not quite right' or they 'don't feel well'.

The information gained from these observations is additional to the safer handling procedure but enables you to fully assess the patient's condition and institute appropriate treatment as necessary, escalating any concerns to senior nurses and the medical team.

☑ **Helpful hints – Do I …?**

- Gloves and aprons must be worn if contact with blood/body fluids/excreta is anticipated or the patient is in isolation.
- Hand hygiene must be performed before touching a patient, before clean/aseptic procedures, after body fluid exposure/risk, after touching a patient and after touching a patient's surroundings.
- Waste should be disposed of in a clinical waste bag if it is contaminated with blood/body fluids/excreta.
- Equipment must be cleaned as identified by the relevant policy every time it is used.

Steps	Reason and patient-centred care considerations
1. The first step of any procedure is to introduce yourself to the patient, explain the procedure and gain their consent.	Fully informed consent may not always be possible if the patient is a child or has mental health illness or learning disabilities, but even in these circumstances, every effort should be made to explain the procedure in terms that the patient can understand. This is not only respectful of their individual human rights, but also helps to ensure that they will be more accepting of the treatment and that their anxieties are reduced. For patients who are unable to provide consent because they are unconscious, advice should be sought from your mentor or another qualified nurse.

Steps	Reason and patient-centred care considerations
2. Gather the equipment required. Ensure this is clean and in working order.	Reduces the chance of infection and maintains patient and nurse safety.
3. Clear sufficient space within the environment, for example around the bed space or chair.	Enables clear access for the patient and the nurse to safely use the equipment required.
4. Wash your hands with soap and water. Apron and gloves should only be worn if appropriate.	Wearing an apron and gloves as part of personal protective equipment (PPE) is a standard infection-control procedure when dealing with body fluids or patients in isolation. Ensure your use of PPE such as gloves and disposable aprons is appropriate by considering the individual patient situation and the risk presented.
5. Close the curtains or take other appropriate measures to maintain the patient's privacy.	Maintain patient privacy, dignity and comfort as required.
6. Position yourself comfortably close to any equipment you are using and adjust the height of beds where possible.	To apply efficient movement principles (see pp. 58–60).
7. The person nearest the head of the patient will lead the move. The move lead must ensure all those in the team understand the requirements of the move and if not, individuals must acknowledge this and step aside.	The move lead takes this position because they can see and communicate with the patient. Moving patients is not just a physical activity but includes interpersonal interaction and is a two-way process between the nurse/move team and the patient to ensure the move is safe and coordinated.
8. All of those involved in moving the patient must be familiar with the handling	Team members must verbally acknowledge to the leader that they are ready, or indeed if they are not.

Steps	Reason and patient-centred care considerations
manoeuvre and agree verbal team commands.	Verbal instructions should include three distinct commands:
	'**Ready**' – allows those involved to prepare a secure starting posture and breath control.
	'**Steady**' – allows those involved to confirm if they are ready to proceed or not.
	'**Move**' – the movement is undertaken.
9. After performing the move ensure the patient is in a comfortable position, with drinks and call bells available as necessary.	Promotes patient comfort and ensures they are well nourished and hydrated.
10. Discard PPE, any single-use equipment and other used materials as per policy. Clean any moving and handling equipment used as per the relevant policy every time it is used and perform hand hygiene.	To prevent cross-infection and maintain equipment in working condition.
11. Document the move and, if necessary, any findings on the patient's observation chart and/ or in the patient's notes.	Maintains patient safety and accurate records.
12. If any abnormalities are observed, escalate to senior nursing staff/ mentor immediately.	It is vital to report abnormal findings to a registered nurse immediately so they can ensure care is escalated. Failure to do so can result in the patient's condition deteriorating, potentially leading to death.

Evidence base: HSE (2000, 2004); Marieb (2013); NMC (2015); Polak (2011); Smith (2011); WHO (2009)

FIRST AID

CHRIS MULRYAN AND CATHERINE DELVES-YATES

The recovery position

☑ **Before you start**
Perform a risk assessment to ensure your safety.

☑ **Field-setting considerations**
You would not put a baby less than one year old in the recovery position; instead, you would simply hold them with their head tilted downwards.

☑ **Care-setting considerations**
A patient can be nursed in the recovery position in any setting.

Steps		Reason and patient-centred care considerations
1.	Perform a head-tilt, chin-lift airway manoeuvre and confirm a clear airway and that the patient is breathing.	To ensure the patient is breathing normally.
2.	Remove any glasses and place the arm nearest to you bent at the elbow out to the side; the so called 'How position'.	To make it easier to roll the patient.
3.	Place the patient's hand (from the opposite side of the body to which you are located) against the patient's face with the palm facing outwards. Place your palm against the patient's.	To support their head.

Steps	Reason and patient-centred care considerations
4. Lift the leg on the opposite side of the body to which you are located at the knee and tuck the foot under the opposite knee.	To assist you to roll the patient.
5. Grasp the patient's hip on the opposite side of the body and roll the patient towards you until they are on their side. Use your knees to control their body movements and your hand to support the head.	Remember to remove any spectacles and any sharp objects from the pockets on the side the person is being rolled on to, to avoid the risk of pressure ulcers developing.
6. Position the bent leg so that it acts as a support.	To reduce the risk of the patient rolling on to their front, which can impair breathing.
7. Position the head using the palm as a support in such a way that secretions or vomit will drain from the airway.	To ensure the airway remains clear.
8. Get help if this has not already been done and monitor the patient's condition.	The patient is now in the recovery position.
9. Document the incident in the patient's notes as appropriate.	Maintains patient safety and accurate records.
10. Ensure incident is reported to senior nursing staff/mentor if they are not already aware.	It is vital to report any abnormal incident to a registered nurse immediately so they can ensure care is escalated. Failure to do so can result in the patient's condition deteriorating, potentially leading to death.

Evidence base: Mulryan (2011); Resuscitation Council (UK) (2010)

ABCDE summary actions

☑ **Before you start**

Perform a risk assessment to ensure your safety.

☑ Field-setting considerations

You can apply Drs ABCDE to any patient in any field.

Cardiac arrest in children is a very rare event. Children's bodies are obviously smaller than those of adults, their physiology is slightly different and the reasons why they become so sick and require resuscitation are often quite different from the causes seen in adults. The techniques required to resuscitate children are different from those used in adults. That said, however, the principles of resuscitation for children mimic those for adults and with a few simple modifications as described in this section, can be applied to children.

☑ Care-setting considerations

You can use Drs ABCDE in any care setting.

Steps	Reason and patient-centred care considerations
1. **D**anger Ensure you are not putting yourself in any danger.	You will not be able to assist the injured person if you also become injured.
2. **R**esponse Assess responsiveness.	To ascertain whether there is anything seriously wrong with the patient, check whether they can respond to you. Ask the patient loudly: 'are you alright?'
3. **S**hout Shout for help.	You will need help in caring for the patient if they are seriously ill, so you need to shout for help and then telephone for either an ambulance or the hospital resuscitation team as soon as you know that your patient is seriously ill.
4. **A**irway Assess the airway.	If a patient does not have a patent airway their body will not be able to receive the oxygen it needs, and they will soon die. Assess their airway by looking for obstruction, listening for sounds and feeling for movement of air.
5. **B**reathing Assess the breathing.	If a patient is not breathing regularly they will not be receiving sufficient air to sustain life. Assessment of the patient's airway in the previous step using the 'look, listen, feel' approach will have provided you with information relating to the patient's breathing. Ask yourself: is this person breathing normally? This means that they are breathing regularly, moving sufficient air to sustain life. If the person is not breathing normally, is making occasional gasps or is not breathing at all then you should start artificial ventilation.

Steps	Reason and patient-centred care considerations
6. **C**irculation Assess the circulation.	A patient needs effective cardiac circulation in order to supply their bodily organs with oxygen and nutrients, then to remove waste products, in order to function effectively. Check whether the patient has a carotid pulse **at the same time** as assessing their breathing. If a patient is not breathing it is highly unlikely that they will have a pulse. If the patient does not have a pulse then you should start external chest compressions.
7. **D**isability Assess the neurological system.	A patient needs a fully functioning brain and nervous system for the body to function effectively. Establishing the level of consciousness that a patient is able to maintain is a fundamental part of establishing the level of disability.
8. **E**xposure Assess for other injuries.	Once you have dealt with immediately life-threatening conditions you can go on to look for any other injuries that the person may have. They may not be immediately aware of these, due to their level of consciousness being reduced or the presence of another distracting injury which is causing them so much pain that they have not actually noticed the additional injuries.

Evidence base: Mulryan (2011); Resuscitation Council (UK) (2010)

Management of choking

☑ **Before you start**
Perform a risk assessment to ensure your safety.

☑ **Field-setting considerations**
If the patient who is choking is a child, there are two differences in the procedure. Firstly, the force of any actions should be reduced. Secondly, abdominal thrusts are unsafe in children and chest thrusts should be used in place of abdominal thrusts. Babies can be picked up and placed with their head positioned downwards, supported on your arm. Larger children can be draped across your knee if you are in a stable sitting position. This again will enable the child's head to be positioned downwards.

☑ **Care-setting considerations**

Choking can be managed in any setting.

Steps	Reason and patient-centred care considerations
1. Ask the conscious person: 'are you choking?' If the person confirms this, carry on. If not, look for an alternative cause.	To ensure the person is choking.
2. Assess the severity of the episode. If the person has an effective cough then the incident is likely to be less severe. Encourage the person to cough: this should be sufficient to clear the obstruction.	If the person can cough you need to remain with them offering reassurance, but encouraging them to cough is the most effective way of clearing the obstruction.
3. If there is no coughing or the cough does not appear to be effective then you will need to perform back-slaps. If possible, and if the person is not already in a standing position, stand them up and lean them forwards.	The person requires your assistance to clear the obstruction. This is an effective position for delivering back-slaps.
4. Stand at the side of the patient and place one hand on their chest to support them.	To ensure the patient is safe.
5. Then slap them firmly between the shoulder blades using the heel of your hand. Do this up to five times or until the obstruction is cleared.	To clear the obstruction.
6. If the airway obstruction persists after you have performed five back-slaps then you will need to proceed to perform abdominal thrusts. Stand behind the patient and make a fist using your right hand. Place your fist thumb-side first, halfway between the patient's belly button and the base of the rib cage.	It is necessary to apply the appropriate force to clear the obstruction.

Steps	Reason and patient-centred care considerations
Reach around the patient from the opposite side with your left hand and grasp your fist. Next pull sharply inwards and upwards whilst at the same time bending the person forwards. Again, repeat this up to five times or until the obstruction is released. Keep your head to one side of the patient's, so their head does not hit you as it comes back.	Chest thrusts present an alternative to abdominal thrusts when abdominal thrusts are not possible or unsafe. Obesity in the patient makes abdominal thrusts difficult to perform and pregnancy makes abdominal thrusts unsafe. You would also never perform abdominal thrusts on a child. Chest thrusts are performed in a similar way to abdominal thrusts, the principal differences being that chest thrusts are performed in the middle of the chest and the force applied is inwards more than inwards and upwards, as is the case in abdominal thrusts.
7. If after you have completed the five abdominal thrusts the airway remains obstructed, continue to repeat cycles of five back-slaps with five abdominal thrusts until the airway obstruction is relieved or the patient loses consciousness. If the patient loses consciousness then immediately start cardiopulmonary resuscitation, starting with chest compressions.	This in itself may be effective in clearing the obstruction.
8. Any patient who has undergone either abdominal or chest thrusts should be evaluated by a doctor.	Both of these first aid interventions can cause injury to the individual. This is the case even if the immediate airway compromise has been completely relieved.

Steps	Reason and patient-centred care considerations
9. Document the incident in the patient's notes as appropriate.	Maintains patient safety and accurate records.
10. Ensure the incident is reported to senior nursing staff/mentor if they are not already aware.	It is vital to report any abnormal incident to a registered nurse immediately so they can ensure care is escalated. Failure to do so can result in the patient's condition deteriorating, potentially leading to death.

Evidence base: Mulryan (2011); Resuscitation Council (UK) (2010)

AVPU assessment

In an emergency situation the AVPU scale is a simple way of communicating the level of responsiveness to other care providers in a clear and understandable way.

It needs to be remembered however, that the AVPU scale does not record subtle changes in a person's mental state which may be an early sign that a person's health is deteriorating. There is quite a significant difference between a person who is alert and a person who is only responsive to voice. More complex methods, such as the Glasgow Coma Scale (GCS) would be used to assess a person's level of consciousness when a more detailed assessment was required.

☑ **Before you start**
If an AVPU assessment is being undertaken in a first aid situation, perform a risk assessment to ensure your safety.

☑ **Field setting considerations**
You can apply AVPU to all patients from all fields as it is a rapid and simple method for assessing neurological status so you can gain initial information about a patient's level of consciousness/responsiveness. If the patient does have a reduced level of consciousness/responsiveness however, you will need to undertake further neurological assessment. This could be with the Glasgow

Coma Scale for adults or a modified paediatric coma score assessment for infants and children.

☑ Care setting considerations
You can use AVPU in any care setting.

☑ What to watch out for and action to take
If the person has a reduced level of responsiveness, scoring V, P or U, or their level of response has altered since it was last assessed report your concerns straight away to your mentor or another registered nurse.

If the patient has a reduced level of consciousness following trauma always consider whether there may be spinal injury and ensure the cervical spine is immobilized.

The information gained from an AVPU assessment will enable you to rapidly assess a person's condition, institute appropriate treatment as necessary and communicate care needs with senior nurses and the medical team.

Steps	Reason and patient-centred care considerations
1. **A** – Assess for alertness by noticing as you approach the person whether they have their eyes open, are interacting with their surroundings and aware of things going on around them. If the person does this, they are 'A' on the AVPU scale.	Healthy people will normally be alert. This means that their eyes will focus on you as you approach and will follow you as you move. Being alert means that a person is reacting and interacting with their environment appropriately, which takes only seconds to assess. Being alert does not mean that the person knows where they are, understands what is going on and knows the date/time. This is described as being 'orientated' and is not part of an AVPU assessment.
2. **V** – If the person is not alert you need to assess for their responsiveness to voice. Ask the patient loudly, 'Are you alright?'	We use the AVPU scale to describe the response that the person maintains. So, if for example a person was not alert when you approached them (because they were asleep), but were woken up by your voice and following this remained alert you should describe them as A. If, however, a person was not alert when you approached them (because they were asleep), but were woken up by your voice and then kept going back to sleep and only responded to your voice, you should described them as V.

Steps	Reason and patient-centred care considerations
If the person responds, they are 'V' on the AVPU scale.	Consider whether it is necessary to place the person in the recovery position (see pp. 64–65), if it is safe to do so, to ensure their airway remains clear.
3. **P** - If the person does not respond to your voice, no matter how loudly you speak to them, you need to assess for their responsiveness to pain. Acceptable ways to assess this are by: a. side finger pressure – squeezing the sides of a finger b. squeezing the trapezius muscle in the neck c. applying pressure over the supraorbital ridge in the eye brow. If the person responds, they are 'P' on the AVPU scale.	Place your thumb at the front of the neck and first finger at the back of the neck. Using a pinching action apply a firm squeeze. Place your thumb below the eyebrow and press firmly. Before attempting either of these techniques with another person, perform them on yourself. This will enable you to gage the correct amount of pressure you need to apply. It is necessary for the pressure you apply to feel acutely uncomfortable, but should not produce extreme amounts of pain. It is never acceptable to inflict extreme pain or use any method to assess for a response to pain that would cause bruising. When assessing for a response to pain, you may find that the person responds immediately to the tactile stimuli of you making physical contact with them. In this case it would not be necessary to perform side finger pressure, a trapezius muscle squeeze or supraorbital ridge pressure. Observe the person closely for any response, which may range from flickering of the eyelids or twitching of facial muscles, to more obvious bodily movement. Place the person in the recovery position (see pp. 64–65), if it is safe to do so, to ensure their airway remains clear.
4. **U** - if the person does not respond to pain in the previous step, they are 'U' on the AVPU scale.	Place the person in the recovery position, if it is safe to do so, to ensure their airway remains clear.

Evidence base: Caton-Richards (2010); Dawes et al. (2007); Mulryan (2011); Resuscitation Council (UK) (2010); Waterhouse (2009)

MEDICINES ADMINISTRATION

CAROL HALL AND CATHERINE DELVES-YATES

Administering medication (oral or topical route)

☑ **Essential equipment**

Drug to be administered

Medication pots (or suitable vessel) to take the drug to the patient in

Jug of water and clean glasses

Medicine Administration Record (MAR)

☑ **Field-specific considerations**

When caring for patients it is important to remember that many have needs which cross the boundaries of the fields of nursing, so consider all of this information as potentially relevant to the patients you may care for.

It is important at all times to empower all patients with respect to medicine administration.

Learning disability – Ensure that the patient and their main carers, as appropriate, are informed about their medicine and about how it assists them. To do this you need to undertake an assessment of the individual's capability. Some people with a learning disability will be able to manage their own medications, whilst others may need varying amounts of support. The use of preloaded and timed pill boxes may be useful in some cases to establish a regular routine and to ensure that your patient takes the correct medicine. Medication administration records which include a photograph of the individual are frequently used in community settings as they provide a safe method of identifying an individual (as identity bands are unlikely to be worn). Another method can be the use of two identifiers (for instance, name and date of birth as well as photo or ID band).

Mental health – The use of physical and psychological supportive techniques and a good understanding of how your patient feels about their medications will assist you in appreciating the extent to which monitoring of medications and support is required. Remember that some patients will be receiving treatment under the Mental Health Act, so may not wish to comply with this. It is also important to consider different models of health belief and self-care in establishing the best care possible for your patient. The therapeutic relationship you have with your patient will influence the information they share in respect of their drug treatment. Remember that other forms of treatment, such as psychotherapy, counselling or cognitive behavioural therapies, may be in effect simultaneously with medication. For some patients with mental health problems, including those who are severely depressed or with suicidal tendencies, when administering medicines you must ensure any medicines given to your patient have been taken. It is important to be aware that medicines may be hidden in the mouth and then secretly stockpiled.

Child – Encourage, assist and educate children of all ages, as well as their parents or carers, to be involved in administration of medicines. This will enable you to determine the capabilities the child may have, their likely behaviour and their understanding of the situation. Ensure you tailor your communication skills to reflect the needs of the different age groups. An awareness of pharmacology and calculation skills to work out patient-specific drug doses is necessary in all fields, but as many drug dosages are determined by a child's weight in kilogrammes it is essential in this field of nursing. It is important that any medication administration is always undertaken away from 'safe' areas, such as the playroom or bedside, especially if the medicine administration is unpleasant.

Adult – In adult nursing all of the above might apply, and your role involves assessing a diverse range of individuals who need your care. Whilst most adults will be able to actively participate in their treatment, you will certainly encounter patients with dementia and those who are confused.

☑ Care-setting considerations
It is possible for medications to be administered orally or topically in all care settings.

☑ What to watch out for and action to take
Monitor effectiveness of the treatment by pre- and post-administration observations. For example, has the patient's temperature reduced; is the patient still in pain or feeling nauseous following administration of medication?

Ensure you are aware of the therapeutic application of the medicine to be administered, its normal dosage, side effects, precautions and contraindications before you administer it. Ensure you refer to an up-to-date version of the British National Formulary (BNF) to ascertain this information before administering any medicines with which you are unfamiliar.

Monitor for any reactions to the medication, report any concerns to your mentor or a registered nurse and ensure they report this to the person prescribing the drug without delay. All drug reactions need to be treated appropriately as soon as they become apparent.

Contact the person prescribing the drug if an assessment of the patient indicates that the medicine is no longer suitable or the patient declines to take it.

☑ **Helpful hints – do I …?**

- Gloves and aprons must be worn if contact with blood/body fluids/excreta is anticipated or the patient is in isolation.
- Gloves should be worn if contact with the medication is potentially harmful to the nurse – for example, in the case of topical steroid preparations.
- Hand hygiene must be performed before touching a patient, before clean/aseptic procedures, after body fluid exposure/risk, after touching a patient and after touching a patient's surroundings.
- Waste should be disposed of in a clinical waste bag if it is contaminated with blood/body fluids/excreta.

Step	Reason and patient-centred care considerations
Ensuring safe and effective storage and administration of medication to patients.	
1. The first step in any procedure is to introduce yourself to the patient, explain the procedure and gain their consent. Ensure that you adapt your communication style to meet the needs of the individual patient and their family or carers as relevant.	Fully informed consent may not always be possible if the patient is a child or has mental health problems or learning disabilities, but even in these circumstances, every effort should be made to explain the procedure in terms that the patient can understand. This is not only respectful of their individual human rights, but also helps to ensure that they will be more accepting of the treatment and that their anxieties are reduced. All patients should be offered the opportunity to be involved in decisions relating to their medicines at their desired level. For patients who are unable to provide consent because they are unconscious, advice should be sought from your mentor or another qualified nurse.

Step	Reason and patient-centred care considerations
2. Gather the equipment required. Ensure it is clean as appropriate.	Reduces the chances of infection and maintains patient and nurse safety.
3. Clear sufficient space within the environment where the drug will be administered.	Enables clear access for the patient and the nurse to safely administer the medication.
4. Wash your hands with soap and water before you start administering medication. Apron and gloves should only be worn if appropriate.	Wearing an apron and gloves as part of personal protective equipment (PPE) is a standard infection-control procedure when dealing with body fluids or patients in isolation. When administering medications it is possible that you may need to wear gloves to protect yourself from exposure to the drug, such as when applying topical skin preparations. Ensure your use of PPE such as gloves and disposable aprons is appropriate by considering the individual patient situation and the risk presented.
5. Patients need to be in a comfortable position, either sitting in a chair, resting on a couch or in bed, as is appropriate.	To promote patient comfort and reduce anxiety.
6. Remember that as a nursing student you need to be supervised by a registered nurse at all times when administering medication.	To ensure patient safety and support your learning.
7. Identify an appropriate place to check and prepare the patient's medications, away from interruptions and distractions.	To ensure patient safety, as interruption is associated with medication error.

Step	Reason and patient-centred care considerations

8. Before you give any medication, you will need to complete a full assessment of your patient's medication needs. This involves:
 	
   a. Checking the patient's care plan for specific requirements.
 	
   b. Checking the Medicine Administration Record (MAR) to determine the correct medicine to be given to the correct patient, taking account of all eight rights of medicine administration.
	To ensure patient safety.
	
	You need to be aware of the patient's plan of care to ensure no changes have been made and that the medication administration remains appropriate.
	
	To ensure the drug is administered accurately and safely.
	
	Medicines must be given in a timely manner in order to ensure optimum benefits from treatments.
	
	It is dangerous to administer a medication which is not specifically licensed for a particular route.

9. If a number of medicines need to be given at the same time, prioritize which one to start with.	If the medications are all to be administered orally it will be possible to take them to the patient at the same time. However, if medication is required via different routes (e.g. injection and oral) at the same time, then this will need to be managed to enable optimum treatment, as some medicines require specific timing or conditions for best effect.
10. Decide if there is any reason not to administer the medicine at this time and record and report accordingly.	If there has been a change in the patient's condition a medication may no be longer appropriate, or the patient may be unable to take it. If a patient is 'nil by mouth', check with the drug prescriber whether any of their oral drugs still need to be given (for example cardiac drugs), possibly by a different route.
11. Locate medicine to be administered and ensure it is:	The quality of an out-of-date medicine may have deteriorated.

Step	Reason and patient-centred care considerations
a. in date	To prevent error and ensure the best possible outcome in terms of patient care.
b. the correct formulation for the route to be given and appropriate for your patient's preferences	To ensure safe practice, as medicines are available in different strengths.
c. the correct dose strength for the prescription	You must check that the prescription and the label on the medicine are both clearly written and are the same to ensure patient safety.
d. the correct medicine according to the prescription	You must never give a medicine without being certain that the dosage (relating to the patient's weight where appropriate), the method of administration, the route and the timing are all correct.
12. If your patient is a child or the drug dose has been calculated taking account of the patient's weight, check that the prescribed dose is correct for the patient's current weight or BMI.	Children's medicines are calculated on the basis of milligrams per kilogramme per day. Some adult drugs are prescribed at a dose which takes account of the patient's weight. To ensure patient safety the dose must be checked, using an accurate patient weight. Some specialized children's areas use BMI and surface area for drug doses. A calculator for this can be found on the BNF website.
13. Calculate the amount of medicine you must give.	An accurate amount of medication must be given to the patient. Medicine must always be measured accurately using appropriate equipment. For example, measuring a dose of 5 ml using a 50 ml medicine pot makes accuracy difficult. With many drugs the difference of even a few mls can cause problems. Always use the smallest appropriate measuring device.

Step	Reason and patient-centred care considerations
14. Ensure the medication is placed into an appropriate receptacle for administration to the patient.	To make taking the medicine as easy as possible for the patient.
15. Medication which is not needed must be returned to its place of secure storage or disposed of in accordance with local policy and legal requirements.	Safe disposal of medicine is important to keep patients, families, carers and, indeed, staff safe from unwanted effects. Controlled medicines and highly toxic materials will have specific guidelines by which you must abide.
16. Complete final checks, which always include patient identity and allergies, but may also include specific checks for individual drugs. Provide patients with necessary information regarding their medication, using appropriate means of communication to aid explanation.	To ensure patient safety: a. you must be certain of the identity of the patient to whom the medicine is to be administered. b. check that the patient is not allergic to the medicine before administering it. c. before administering some drugs, cardiac ones for example, it is necessary to check that the patient's heart rate or blood pressure is not too low. Patients and their families and carers need to be aware of the main features of the medicines given and how to manage them effectively and concordantly. They need to know what to do if the medicine is taken inappropriately and the implications of not taking it.
17. Ensure your patient is fully prepared for the administration of the medication and is in an appropriate position. Provide protective clothing or tissues if needed, or a drink, etc. An infant may need to be held securely.	Patients should be in a position which ensures both comfort and safety. Protective clothing can maintain dignity through avoiding spills.

Step	Reason and patient-centred care considerations
18. Ensure medication is administered in accordance with the prescription, local policy and patient preferences. If given orally, ensure medication has been swallowed.	To ensure patient safety and involvement.

Recording administration and outcome

1. Record that the medicine has been administered on the Medication Administration Record to ensure a legal record of the medicine administered.	You must make a clear, accurate and immediate record of all medicine administered, or any intentionally withheld or refused by the patient. You must ensure your signature is clear and legible. Ensure the registered nurse supervising you countersigns your signature.

Evaluation of the impact and effectiveness of the medication and assessment of any untoward events

1. Monitor the effectiveness of the medication and any reactions, reporting these to a registered nurse and the medication prescriber and instigating treatment as appropriate.	Ensure you are fully aware of the therapeutic uses of the medicine to be administered, its normal dosage, side effects, precautions and contraindications. Adverse reactions to medications can range from discomforting to life-threatening. By administering a medicine you undertake to ensure that you are aware of any possible reactions and know what to do in response. Ensure you advise patients of any signs to watch out for and identify how they can inform you.

Step	Reason and patient-centred care considerations
2. After the medication administration has been completed ensure the patient is in a comfortable position, with drinks and call bells available as necessary.	Promotes patient comfort and ensures they are well nourished and hydrated.
3. Discard PPE, any single-use equipment and other used materials as per policy. Clean any equipment used as per the relevant policy every time it is used and perform hand hygiene.	To prevent cross-infection and maintain equipment in working condition.
4. Document relevant information on the patient's observation chart and/or in the patient's notes as necessary.	Maintains patient safety and accurate records.

Evidence base: BNF (2014); National Prescribing Centre (NPC) (n.d.); NMC (2007, updated 2008, 2009, 2010a); Westbrook et al. (2010); WHO (2009)

Adapted from Hall (2002)

Administering a subcutaneous injection

☑ **Essential equipment**
Drug to be administered, either in a prefilled syringe with a non-detachable needle or in an ampoule, sterile swab (to open ampoule), blunt fill needle (to draw up drug if not using a prefilled syringe, with a filter if drawing up from a glass ampoule), safety needle (to give drug if not using a prefilled syringe, choice depends upon patient and drug to be given), appropriately sized

syringe, injection tray (or similar), gloves, sharps bin, spot plaster (or similar) to cover injection site.

Medicine Administration Record (MAR).

☑ Field specific considerations
Refer to Administering Medications (pp. 75–81).

It is not uncommon for both adults and children to be very worried about having an injection. Make sure you take time to relax the patient as much as is possible and answer any questions they have. The patient may wish to have another person they trust present for the procedure (or it might be necessary to have the assistance of another member of the healthcare team or a play specialist), to hold the patient's hand and distract their attention by, for example, talking, story-telling, singing etc.

Local anaesthetic creams are frequently used prior to subcutaneous administration of medicines in children.

☑ Care setting considerations
It is possible for a subcutaneous injection to be administered in all care settings.

☑ What to watch out for and action to take
Refer to Administering Medications (pp. 75–81).

Subcutaneous injections are given in to the fatty layer of tissue just under the skin. As blood flow to fatty tissue is relatively poor, any medication given by this route will be absorbed slowly, sometimes taking up to 24 hours.

Never give a subcutaneous injection into skin that is burned, hardened, inflamed, swollen or damaged by a previous injection.

There are a number of sites where subcutaneous injections are frequently given. The site chosen will depend upon the volume of medication to be given and how thick it is, plus the amount of subcutaneous tissue the patient has at the injection site. The site to be used should be decided upon after consideration of these factors and take into account the patient's preference. When a patient is receiving regular subcutaneous injections it is important to rotate the site, to prevent scarring and hardening of the tissue.

Do not give a subcutaneous injection within 5cm of the navel or any scar tissue.

It is not necessary to decontaminate socially clean skin with an alcohol wipe prior to administering a subcutaneous injection as alcohol causes the skin to harden, which will alter absorption of the medication when the site is next used.

If the skin is visibly soiled decontamination using an alcohol wipe is appropriate.

When administering an injection ensure that you always adhere to all of the relevant policies outlined by the healthcare provider and your educational institution.

☑ **Helpful Hints – Do I…?**

- Gloves and aprons must be worn if contact with blood/body fluids/excreta is anticipated or the patient is in isolation.
- Gloves must be worn for all invasive procedures and all activities carrying a risk of exposure to blood, body fluids, or to sharp or contaminated instruments.
- Gloves should be worn if contact with the medication is potentially harmful to the nurse.
- Hand hygiene must be performed before touching a patient, before clean/aseptic procedures, after body fluid exposure/risk, after touching a patient and after touching a patient's surroundings.
- Waste should be disposed of in a clinical waste bag if it is contaminated with blood/body fluids/excreta.

Step	Reason and patient-centred care considerations
Ensuring safe and effective storage and administration of medication to patients.	
1. Remember that as a nursing student you need to be supervised at all times by a registered nurse when administering medication.	To ensure patient safety and support your learning.
2. Identify an appropriate place to check the patient's medication, away from interruptions and distractions.	To ensure patient safety as interruption is associated with medication error.
3. Before you give any medication you will need to complete an assessment of your patient's medication needs. This involves: a. Checking the patient's care plan for specific requirements.	To ensure patient safety. You need to be aware of the patient's plan of care to ensure no changes have been made and that the medication administration remains appropriate. To ensure the drug is administered accurately and safely.

Step	Reason and patient-centred care considerations
b. Checking the Medicine Administration Record (MAR) to determine the correct medicine to be given by subcutaneous injection to the correct patient, taking account of all 8 rights of medicine administration.	Medicines must be given in a timely manner in order to ensure optimum benefits from treatments. It is dangerous to administer a medication which does not have a specific licence for a particular route.
4. Decide if there is any reason not to administer the subcutaneous injection at this time and record and report accordingly.	If there has been a change in the patient's condition a medication may no longer be appropriate.
5. Ensure the drug to be administered by subcutaneous injection is: a. in date. b. the correct dose for the prescription. c. the correct medicine according to the prescription.	The quality of an out of date medicine may have deteriorated To prevent error and ensure the best possible outcome in terms of patient care. To ensure safe practice as medicines are available in different strengths. You must check that the prescription is clearly written and the medication is the same to ensure patient safety. You must never give a medicine without being certain that the dosage (relating to the patient's weight where appropriate), the method of administration, the route and the timing are all correct.
6. If your patient is a child or the drug dose has been calculated taking account of the patient's weight, check that the prescribed dose is correct for the patient's current weight or BMI.	Children's medicines are calculated on the basis of milligrams per kilogramme per day. Some adult drugs are prescribed at a dose which takes account of the patient's weight. To ensure patient safety the dose must be checked, using an accurate patient weight.

Step	Reason and patient-centred care considerations
	Some specialized children's areas use BMI and surface area for drug doses. A calculator for this can be found for this in the BNF for children online at www.bnf.org.uk.
7. Injections should be prepared in a clean area using an aseptic non-touch technique.	To reduce the risk of infection.
8. If using a prefilled syringe this step is not required as the drug is already in the syringe!	
If drawing up the drug:	
a. Attach a blunt fill needle to the syringe. Make sure you use one with a filter if you are drawing a drug up from a glass ampoule.	To reduce the risk of glass particles being drawn up with the medication.
b. If the drug is in a glass ampoule, flick it to remove any medication from the top.	To ensure all medication is drawn up.
c. Cover the top of the ampoule with a sterile swab and snap it off along the score lines at the neck.	To remove the medication safely from the ampoule.
d. Check that there are no particles of glass in the medication; if there are, use a new ampoule.	To ensure the medication given to the patient does not contain glass.
e. Draw the drug up into the syringe.	To encourage any air bubbles to rise so they can be expelled.
f. Holding the syringe upright, with the needle at the top, tap the side of the syringe.	To leave the correct dose in the syringe
g. Expel the air and any excess medication.	To ensure safety.
h. Remove the fill needle and dispose of it in the sharps bin.	
i. Attach the safety needle to be used to administer the medication using a non-touch technique.	
Either 27G or 31G safety needles are frequently chosen to administer medication subcutaneously.	The choice of needle depends upon the patient's size and the viscosity of the medication.

Step	Reason and patient-centred care considerations
9. Place the syringe containing the medication on an injection tray with a spot plaster and take it to the patient with the Medicines Administration Record (MAR). Ensure a sharps bin is to hand.	To safely dispose of the syringe once the medication has been administered. Fully informed consent may not always be possible if the patient is a child, has mental health problems, or learning disabilities; but even in these circumstances, every effort should be made to explain the procedure in terms that the patient can understand. This is not only respectful of their individual human rights, but also helps to ensure that they will be more accepting of the treatment and that their anxieties are reduced.
10. Introduce yourself to the patient, explain the procedure and gain their consent. Ensure that you adapt your communication style to meet the needs of the individual patient and their family or carers as relevant.	All patients should be offered the opportunity to be involved in decisions relating to their medicines at the level they wish. For patients who are unable to provide consent because they are unconscious advice should be sought.
11. Clear sufficient space within the environment where the drug will be administered. Place the injection tray containing the syringe in a safe place where you can see it at all times.	Enables clear access for the patient and the nurse to safely administer the medication. To ensure patient safety whilst you complete the next step.
12. Complete the final checks, which always include patient identity and allergies but may also include specific checks for individual drugs.	To ensure patient safety you must: a. be certain of the identity of the patient to whom the medicine is to be administered. b. check that the patient is not allergic to the medicine before administering it.

Step	Reason and patient-centred care considerations
Provide patient with necessary information regarding their medication, using appropriate means of communication to aid explanation.	c. before administering some drugs, cardiac ones for example, it is necessary to check that the patient's heart rate or blood pressure is not too low.
	Patients, their families and carers need to be aware of the main features of the medicines given and how to manage them effectively and concordantly. They need to know what to do if the medicine is taken inappropriately and the implications of not taking it.
13. Decide which injection site is going to be used. Ensure your patient is fully prepared for the administration of the subcutaneous injection and is in an appropriate position. An infant may need to be held securely.	Offer the patient the opportunity to be involved in the decision of choice of site as is appropriate. Patients should be in a position which ensures both comfort and safety.
14. Ask and/or assist the patient to remove their clothing as is necessary to expose the injection site.	Ensure you maintain the patient's dignity and privacy.
15. Perform hand hygiene and put on gloves. Remove the cover from the needle of the syringe, taking care not to contaminate it.	To reduce the chance of infection. Gloves must be worn for all invasive procedures and all activities carrying a risk of exposure to blood, body fluids, or to sharp or contaminated instruments. To ensure the needle is not contaminated.
16. Hold the syringe like a pencil in the hand you write with. Ensure the needle is pointing towards the patient. Gently pinch the patient's skin at the chosen site between	Pinching up the skin between your thumb and first finger ensures that the subcutaneous tissue is separated from the muscle below. If the skin is not pinched up, it could result in administering the medication into the muscle rather than the subcutaneous tissue.

Step	Reason and patient-centred care considerations
	the thumb and first finger with your other hand. The fold of pinched skin should be approximately twice as long as the needle.	
17.	Quickly insert the needle all the way into the fold of skin at an angle of 90 degrees, unless a different angle is recommended by the manufacturer. Do not push the needle into the skin slowly or stab the needle into the skin with extreme force.	To minimize the discomfort felt by the patient. Always ensure that you are aware of the specific manufacturer's instructions in relation to how the drug should be injected (angle of needle and site of administration). Not following this advice will mean that you are not abiding by the licence issued for the injection, so you are giving the injection incorrectly and may be exposing the patient to unnecessary risk.
18.	Whilst continuing to keep the skin pinched up, press the syringe plunger down to inject the medication smoothly and slowly, at a rate of 1ml over 10seconds. Once all of the medication has been injected quickly remove the needle and then release the pinched up skin.	To ensure the medication is administered into the subcutaneous tissue. To minimize the discomfort felt by the patient.
19.	As soon as you have removed the needle from the patient, activate the needle safety device, if present, which will automatically cover the needle. Dispose of the needle and syringe in the sharps bin and any	To reduce the chance of accidental needle stick injury. To maintain nurse and patient safety. Some injection sites may leak a very small amount of fluid or blood.

Step	Reason and patient-centred care considerations
	other equipment as per local policy. If necessary cover the injection site with a spot plaster.	
20.	Remove gloves and perform hand hygiene.	To reduce the chance of infection. If PPE is required because the patient is in isolation put on a new pair of gloves.
21.	After the medication administration has been completed ensure the patient is in a comfortable position with drinks and call bells available as necessary.	Promotes patient comfort and ensures they are well nourished and hydrated.
22.	Discard PPE, any single use equipment and other used materials as per policy. Clean any equipment used as per the relevant policy every time it is used and perform hand hygiene.	To prevent cross infection and maintain equipment in working condition.
Recording administration and outcome.	
1.	Record that the medicine has been administered on the Medication Administration Record to ensure a legal record of the medicine administered.	You must make a clear, accurate and immediate record of all medicine administered, or any intentionally withheld or refused by the patient. You must ensure your signature is clear and legible. Ensure the registered nurse supervising you countersigns your signature.
Evaluation of the impact and effectiveness of the medication and assessment of any untoward events.	
1.	Monitor the effectiveness of the medication and any reactions, reporting these to a registered nurse and the medication prescriber and instigating treatment as appropriate.	Ensure you are fully aware of the therapeutic uses of the medicine to be administered, its normal dosage, side effects, precautions and contra-indications.

Step	Reason and patient-centred care considerations
	Adverse reactions to medications can range from giving discomfort to being life threatening. By administering a medicine you undertake to ensure that you are aware of any possible reactions and you know what to do in response. Ensure you advise patients' of any signs to watch out for and identify how they can inform you.
2. Document relevant information on the patient's observation chart and/or in the patient's notes as necessary.	Maintains patient safety and accurate records.

Evidence base: Adapted from Hall (2002)

Administering an intramuscular injection

☑ **Essential equipment**
Drug to be administered, sterile swab (to open ampoule), blunt fill needle (to draw up drug, with a filter if drawing up from a glass ampoule), safety needle (to give drug – often 21G, but choice depends upon patient and drug to be given), appropriately sized syringe, alcohol swab (for skin preparation according to local policy), injection tray (or similar), gloves, sharps bin, gauze (or similar) to apply pressure to injection site, spot plaster (or similar) to cover injection site.
Medicine Administration Record (MAR).

☑ **Field specific considerations**
Refer to Administering Medications (pp. 75–81).

It is not uncommon for both adults and children to be very worried about having an injection. Make sure you take time to relax the patient as much as is possible and answer any questions they have. The patient may wish to have another person they trust present for the procedure (or it might be necessary to have the assistance of another member of the healthcare team or a play specialist), to hold the patient's hand and distract their attention by, for example, talking, story-telling, singing etc.

With children local anaesthetic cream is often applied prior to the procedure. The intramuscular injection route is often used when nursing children, with the exception of immunizations and in emergency situations.

☑ Care setting considerations
It is possible for an intramuscular injection to be administered in all care settings.

☑ What to watch out for and action to take
Refer to Administering Medications (pp. 75–81).

Intramuscular injections are given in to the skeletal muscle. As blood flow to muscle is good, any medication given by this route will be absorbed more rapidly than if it is given orally or by a subcutaneous injection, but not as quickly as an intravenous injection.

When administering an injection ensure that you always adhere to all of the relevant policies outlined by the healthcare provider and your educational institution.

There are four sites that can be used for an intramuscular injection. The site chosen will depend upon the volume of medication to be given and how thick it is, plus the amount of muscle tissue the patient has at the injection site. The site to be used should be decided upon after consideration of these factors and take into account the patient's preference.

Deltoid
A site that is easy to access, but the muscle is small and only suitable for the administration of 1-2mls of drug (depending upon how well developed the muscle is). There is also risk of injury to the axillary nerve in particular, plus other nerves and blood vessels in the area.

Dorsogluteal
This is the most frequently used site in adults, where up to 3mls of drug can be administered.

The dorsogluteal site is contraindicated in children. There is the possibility of causing damage to the sciatic nerve when using this site, which can cause pain or paralysis that may be permanent. The position of the superior gluteal artery also makes inadvertent arterial drug administration a potential risk, as is accidental subcutaneous drug administration if the wrong needle choice is made in patients with larger amounts of subcutaneous tissue.

Tissue necrosis, gangrene, pain, muscle contraction and fibrosis have all been associated with intramuscular injections in this site.

Vastus lateralis

An easy to access site, with few major blood vessels in the area. The site can be used to administer up to 2mls of drug. Using this site can, however, cause pain and the depth of subcutaneous tissue will vary between patients.

Ventogluteal

This site provides the greatest thickness of gluteal muscle which can take up to 3mls of drug. As there are no nerves or blood vessels in this area and the layer of subcutaneous tissue is thin, it is the preferable site for an intramuscular injection. Despite these positive factors however, it is not frequently used in practice in the UK.

The evidence supporting the need to decontaminate the skin prior to administering an intramuscular injection is debated, so ensure that you follow the policy of the healthcare provider. If alcohol swabs are used, ensure you leave the site to dry, as alcohol can inactivate medication.

☑ Helpful Hints – Do I ...?

- Gloves and aprons must be worn if contact with blood/body fluids/excreta is anticipated or the patient is in isolation.
- Gloves must be worn for all invasive procedures and all activities carrying a risk of exposure to blood, body fluids, or to sharp or contaminated instruments.
- Gloves should be worn if contact with the medication is potentially harmful to the nurse.
- Hand hygiene must be performed before touching a patient, before clean/aseptic procedures, after body fluid exposure/risk, after touching a patient and after touching a patient's surroundings.
- Waste should be disposed of in a clinical waste bag if it is contaminated with blood/body fluids/excreta.

Step	Reason and patient-centred care considerations
Ensuring safe and effective storage and administration of medication to patients.	
1. Remember that as a nursing student you need to be supervised at all times by a registered nurse when administering medication.	To ensure patient safety and support your learning.
2. Identify an appropriate place to check the patient's medication, away from interruptions and distractions.	To ensure patient safety as interruption is associated with medication error.
3. Before you give any medication you will need to complete an assessment of your patient's medication needs. This involves:	To ensure patient safety.
a. Checking the patient's care plan for specific requirements.	You need to be aware of the patient's plan of care to ensure no changes have been made and that the medication administration remains appropriate.
b. Checking the Medicine Administration Record (MAR) to determine the correct medicine to be given by intramuscular injection to the correct patient, taking account of all 8 rights of medicine administration.	To ensure the drug is administered accurately and safely. Medicines must be given in a timely manner in order to ensure optimum benefits from treatments. It is dangerous to administer a medication which does not have a specific licence for a particular route.
4. Decide if there is any reason not to administer the intravenous injection at this time and record and report accordingly.	If there has been a change in the patient's condition a medication may no longer be appropriate.

Step	Reason and patient-centred care considerations
5. Ensure the drug to be administered by intramuscular injection is: a. in date. b. the correct dose for the prescription. c. the correct medicine according to the prescription.	The quality of an out of date medicine may have deteriorated. To prevent error and ensure the best possible outcome in terms of patient care. To ensure safe practice as medicines are available in different strengths. You must check that the prescription is clearly written and the medication in is the same to ensure patient safety. You must never give a medicine without being certain that the dosage (relating to the patient's weight where appropriate), the method of administration, the route and the timing are all correct.
6. If your patient is a child or the drug dose has been calculated taking account of the patient's weight, check that the prescribed dose is correct for the patient's current weight or BMI.	Children's medicines are calculated on the basis of milligrams per kilogramme per day. Some adult drugs are prescribed at a dose which takes account of the patient's weight. To ensure patient safety the dose must be checked, using an accurate patient weight. Some specialized children's areas use BMI and surface area for drug doses. A calculator for this can be found for this in the BNF for children online at www.bnf.org.uk.
7. Gather the equipment required, including the needles and a syringe of the appropriate size for the amount of medication to be injected.	To ensure safe administration of the drug and safe disposal of the sharps once the medication has been administered.

Step		Reason and patient-centred care considerations
8.	Wash your hands with soap and water. Apron and gloves should only be worn if appropriate.	It may be necessary to wear gloves and an apron during the preparation of some medications.
		Wearing apron and gloves as part of personal protective equipment (PPE) is a standard infection control procedure when dealing with body fluids or patients in isolation.
		Ensure your use of PPE such as gloves and disposable aprons is appropriate by considering the individual patient situation and the risk presented.
9.	Injections should be prepared in a clean area using an aseptic non-touch technique.	To reduce the risk of infection.
	Attach a blunt fill needle to the syringe. Make sure you use one with a filter if you are drawing a drug up from a glass ampoule.	To reduce the risk of glass particles being drawn up with the medication.
10.	If the drug is in a glass ampoule, flick it to remove any medication from the top.	To ensure all medication is drawn up from the ampoule.
	Cover the top of the ampoule with a sterile swab and snap it off along the score lines at the neck.	To remove the medication safely from the ampoule.
	Check that there are no particles of glass in the medication, if there are, use a new ampoule.	To ensure the medication given to the patient does not contain glass.

Step		Reason and patient-centred care considerations
11.	Draw the medication up into the syringe.	To encourage any air bubbles to rise so they can be expelled.
	Holding the syringe upright, with the needle at the top, tap the side of the syringe.	
	Expel the air and any excess medication, leaving the correct dose in the syringe.	
12.	Remove the fill needle and dispose of it in the sharps bin.	To ensure safety.
	Attach the safety needle to be used to administer the medication using a non-touch technique.	A 21G safety needle (normally green) is frequently chosen to administer medication intramuscularly. The choice however will depend upon the size of the patient and how viscous the medication is.
13.	Place the syringe on the injection tray with the other equipment and take it to the patient with the Medicines Administration Record (MAR). Ensure a sharps bin is to hand.	To enable safe administration of the medication and safe disposal of sharps.
14.	Introduce yourself to the patient, explain the procedure and gain their consent.	Fully informed consent may not always be possible if the patient is a child, has mental health problems, or learning disabilities; but even in these circumstances, every effort should be made to explain the procedure in terms that the patient can understand. This is not only respectful of their individual human rights, but also helps to ensure that they will be more accepting of the treatment and that their anxieties are reduced.
	Ensure that you adapt your communication style to meet the needs of the individual patient and their family or carers as relevant.	

Step	Reason and patient-centred care considerations
	All patients should be offered the opportunity to be involved in decisions relating to their medicines at the level they wish.
	For patients who are unable to provide consent because they are unconscious advice should be sought.
15. Clear sufficient space within the environment where the drug will be administered.	Enables clear access for the patient and the nurse to safely administer the medication.
Place the injection tray containing the syringe in a safe place where you can see it at all times.	To ensure patient safety whilst you complete the next step.
16. Complete the final checks, which always include patient identity and allergies but may also include specific checks for individual drugs. Provide the patient with necessary information regarding their medication, using appropriate means of communication to aid explanation.	To ensure patient safety you must: a. be certain of the identity of the patient to whom the medicine is to be administered. b. check that the patient is not allergic to the medicine before administering it. c. before administering some drugs, cardiac ones for example, it is necessary to check that the patient's heart rate or blood pressure is not too low. Patients, their families and carers need to be aware of the main features of the medicines given and how to manage them effectively and concordantly. They need to know what to do if the medicine is taken inappropriately and the implications of not taking it.

Step	Reason and patient-centred care considerations		
17. Decide which injection site is to be used.	Offer the patient the opportunity to be involved in this decision as is appropriate.		
Ensure the patient is fully prepared for the administration of the intramuscular injection and is in an appropriate position (see next step). An infant may need to be held securely.	Patients should be in a position which ensures both comfort and safety.		
Ask and/or assist the patient to remove their clothing as is necessary to expose the injection site (see next step).	Ensure you maintain the patient's dignity and privacy.		

	Deltoid Site	Dorsogluteal Site	Vastus lateralis Site	Ventrogluteal Site
18.	Seat the patient, although they may wish to stand.	Position the patient lying on their side to expose the chosen buttock.	Position the patient lying on their back. May also be given in the sitting position, which may reflect patient preference.	Position the patient either lying on their back or side, or they may wish to stand.	To ensure patient is in a comfortable position that enables access to the chosen site.
19.	To make it easier to locate the deltoid muscle expose the patient's arm and shoulder, asking them to place their arm across their	To make it easier to locate the dorsogluteal muscle ask the patient to bend up their knees.	To make it easier to locate the vastus lateralis muscle expose the patient's leg.	To make it easier to locate the ventrogluteal muscle ask the patient to bend up their knee on the chosen side.	

Step	Reason and patient-centred care considerations
20. Locate the exact injection site.	To ensure injection is given into muscle identified.
21. Perform hand hygiene and put on gloves.	To reduce the chance of infection.
	Gloves must be worn for all invasive procedures and all activities carrying a risk of exposure to blood, body fluids, or to sharp or contaminated instruments.
22. Remove the cover from the needle of the syringe, taking care not to contaminate it.	To ensure the needle is not contaminated.
23. Hold the syringe like a pencil in the hand you write with. Ensure the needle is pointing towards the patient.	This technique is known as Z-tracking, which reduces pain and leaking from the injection site.
Use the thumb of your other hand to stretch the skin over the injection site by 2 to 3 cm.	You may see variations in the practice of registered nurses – some will use z tracking and others may not. It is always important to ensure that you follow the drug manufacturer's recommendations and are aware of the relevant research evidence. In this way you can be certain that you give the injection correctly.
24. Whilst continuing to stretch the skin, quickly insert the needle all the way into the skin at an angle of 90 degrees. Do not push the needle into the skin slowly or stab the needle into the skin with extreme force.	To minimize the discomfort felt by the patient.
	To ensure the muscle is reached and the medication is not administered into the subcutaneous tissue.

Step	Reason and patient-centred care considerations
25. Whilst continuing to stretch the skin, if you are using the dorsogluteal site, check for any 'flashback', by pulling back on the plunger of the syringe.	Flashback describes blood entering the syringe. It is not necessary to do this with the deltoid or vastus lateralis sites, as there a few major blood vessels in these areas.
If blood enters the syringe, withdraw the needle and start the procedure again.	If blood is drawn back into the syringe the needle is in a blood vessel and if you administered the medication it would enter the blood supply.
There is no need to undertake this step with the deltoid, vastus lateralis or ventrogluteal site.	These sites do not have the risk of the needle entering a blood vessel.
26. Whilst continuing to stretch the skin, slowly press the syringe plunger down to inject the medication smoothly and slowly at a rate of 1ml per 10 seconds.	To minimize the discomfort felt by the patient. Administering the medication slowly will allow the muscle fibres to stretch in order to make space for the fluid being injected.
27. Whilst continuing to stretch the skin, once all of the medication has been injected, wait 10 seconds before quickly removing the needle.	This allows the medication to disperse evenly.
When the needle has been removed, release the stretch being applied to the skin.	Releasing the stretch is the final part of the Z-tracking process, which prevents the fluid from leaking out of the injection site.
28. As soon as you have removed the needle from the patient, activate the needle safety device, if present, which will automatically cover the needle.	To reduce the chance of accidental needle stick injury.

Step	Reason and patient-centred care considerations
Dispose of the needle and syringe in the sharps bin and any other equipment as per local policy.	To maintain nurse and patient safety.
If necessary apply pressure to the injection site with dry gauze and cover with a spot plaster.	Some injection sites may leak a very small amount of fluid or blood.
29. Remove gloves and perform hand hygiene.	To reduce the chance of infection.
	If PPE is required because the patient is in isolation put on a new pair of gloves.
30. After the medication administration has been completed ensure the patient is in a comfortable position with drinks and call bells available as necessary.	Promotes patient comfort and ensures they are well nourished and **hydrated**.
31. Discard PPE, any single use equipment and other used materials as per policy. Clean any equipment used as per the relevant policy every time it is used and perform hand hygiene.	To prevent cross infection and maintain equipment in working condition.
Recording administration and outcome.	
1. Record that the medicine has been administered on the Medication Administration Record to ensure a legal record of the medicine administered.	You must make a clear, accurate and immediate record of all medicine administered, or any intentionally withheld or refused by the patient. You must ensure your signature is clear and legible. Ensure the registered nurse supervising you countersigns your signature.

Step	Reason and patient-centred care considerations
Evaluation of the impact and effectiveness of the medication and assessment of any untoward events.	
1. Monitor the effectiveness of the medication and any reactions, reporting these to a registered nurse and the medication prescriber and instigating treatment as appropriate.	Ensure you are fully aware of the therapeutic uses of the medicine to be administered, its normal dosage, side effects, precautions and contra-indications.
	Adverse reactions to medications can range from giving discomfort to being life threatening. By administering a medicine you undertake to ensure that you are aware of any possible reactions and you know what to do in response.
	Ensure you advise patients of any signs to watch out for and identify how they can inform you.
2. Document relevant information on the patient's observation chart and/or in the patient's notes as necessary.	Maintains patient safety and accurate records.

Evidence base: Baillie (2009); BNF (2014); Cocoman and Murray (2007, 2008); Dougherty and Lister (2011); National Prescribing Centre (n.d.); NICE (2012a); NMC (2007, 2010); NMC (2012a); RCN (2011a); Westbrook et al. (2010) WHO (2009, 2014)

Adapted from Hall (2002)

ASSISTING PATIENTS WITH THEIR NUTRITIONAL NEEDS

KATE GOODHAND AND JANE EWEN

Common steps for all nutrition-related skills

☑ **Essential equipment**

Depends upon skill but is likely to include one or more of the following: utensils, crockery with or without adaptations, plate guard, slip mat, napkin/disposable clothes protection.

☑ **Field-specific considerations**

When caring for a patient with a learning disability it is important to know their level of understanding so that consent for and cooperation with the care can be gained. You will need to allow time to explain what you are doing and whether it will cause discomfort or pain.

Patients who have mental health problems may not understand why you need to undertake nutrition-related skills. They may also be so depressed that they don't have the energy to eat, or those with cognitive impairment may have forgotten to eat. They may withhold consent to have their measurements taken and you may need to refer to the Mental Capacity Act 2005 and best interest.

Children have different anatomy and physiology to adults, which varies from birth through to adolescence. You will need knowledge of paediatric anatomy and physiology to enable you to interpret the results. As younger children may not understand why you need to undertake the skill, you will need to modify your approach. It is usually helpful to have the parents or carers present to assist.

☑ **Care-setting considerations**

In hospital or care homes, seek the patient's preference for eating alone or in company. At home individuals may need food and drink prepared and served by healthcare workers.

☑ What to watch out for and action to take

Whilst undertaking any nutrition-related skill, you should also assess:

- the position of the patient;
- their neurological condition – are they alert and responsive?;
- any signs or complaints of pain or discomfort;
- the patient's or relative's views – these may provide you with important additional information.

The information gained from these observations will enable you to fully assess the patient's condition, institute appropriate treatment as necessary and escalate needs care to senior nurses and the medical team.

☑ Helpful hints – Do I ...?

- Gloves and aprons must be worn if the patient is in isolation.
- Hand hygiene must be performed before touching a patient, after touching a patient and after touching a patient's surroundings.
- Waste should be disposed of in a clinical waste bag.

Step	Reason and patient-centred care considerations
1. The first step of any procedure is to introduce yourself to the patient, explain the procedure and gain their consent.	Fully informed consent may not always be possible if the patient is a child or has mental health problems or learning disabilities, but even in these circumstances, every effort should be made to explain the procedure in terms that the patient can understand. This is not only respectful of their individual human rights, but also helps to ensure that they will be more accepting of the treatment and that their anxieties are reduced. For patients who are unable to provide consent because they are unconscious, advice should be sought from your mentor or a qualified nurse.
2. Gather the equipment required (see individual skills for equipment required). Ensure these are clean and in working order.	Reduces the chance of infection and maintains patient and nurse safety.

Step	Reason and patient-centred care considerations
3. Clear sufficient space within the environment, for example around the bed space or chair.	Enables clear access for the patient and the nurse to safely use the equipment required.
4. Wash your hands with soap and water before you start the skill. Apron and gloves should only be worn if appropriate.	Wearing an apron and gloves as part of personal protective equipment (PPE) is a standard infection-control procedure when a patient is in isolation. Ensure your use of PPE such as gloves and disposable aprons is appropriate by considering the individual patient situation and the risk presented.
5. Ask the patient if they wish to have the curtains drawn for privacy or to be in a separate room.	Some patients may feel exposed. Maintain patient privacy, dignity and comfort as required.
6. Patients need to be in a comfortable position, either sitting in a chair, resting on a couch or in bed.	To promote patient comfort and reduce anxiety.
7. After performing the skill ensure the patient is in a comfortable position, with drinks and call bells available as necessary.	Promotes patient comfort and ensures they are well nourished and hydrated.
8. Discard PPE, any single-use equipment and other used materials as per policy. Clean any equipment used as per the relevant policy every time it is used and perform hand hygiene.	To prevent cross-infection and maintain equipment in working condition.
9. Document findings on the patient's observation chart and/or in the patient's notes.	Maintains patient safety and accurate records.
10. If any changes are observed, escalate to senior nursing staff/mentor immediately.	It is vital to report changes to a registered nurse immediately so they can ensure care is escalated.

Evidence base: Dougherty and Lister (2011); WHO (2009)

Weighing a patient (Wt)

☑ What is normal
Most adults will know their height but often get their weight wrong!

Refer to BMI chart to determine if weight is in proportion to height.

☑ Before you start
Remember the common steps for all nutrition-related skills (pp. 104–105).

☑ Essential equipment
Appropriate weighing scales:
- 0–2 years – baby scales
- Over 2 years sitting or standing scales
- For patients with mobility needs – hoist scales

☑ Field-specific considerations
When caring for a patient with a learning disability it is important to know their level of understanding so that consent for and cooperation with the measurement can be gained. You will need to allow time to explain what you are doing and why.

Patients who have mental health problems may not understand why you need to undertake nutrition-related skills, or may simply require further details, full explanation and reassurance.

If you are weighing a child prepare them using an age-appropriate explanation (you may use a play specialist to assist). If possible, involve the child's parents or carers to reassure the child. If a child becomes upset do not weigh them, but document the reason and return later.

☑ Care-setting considerations
Patients can be weighed in any care setting, as long as the scales are in working order and accurately calibrated.

☑ What to watch out for and action to take
Whilst undertaking any nutrition-related skill, you should also assess:

- the patient's positioning and ability to mobilize;
- their neurological condition – are they alert and responsive?
- any signs or complaints of pain or discomfort;
- the patient's or relatives' views, as these may provide you with important additional information.

The information gained from these observations will enable you to fully assess the patient's condition, institute appropriate treatment as necessary and escalate needs care to senior nurses and the medical team.

Step	Reason and patient-centred care considerations
1. Perform steps 1-6 of the common steps (pp. 104-105).	To prepare the patient and yourself to undertake the skill.
2. Remove clothing as appropriate: • 0-2 remove clothing. • Over 2 remove shoes or slippers and empty pockets.	Reduces the chance of abnormal readings.
3. Ensure scales are on flat surface and the dial is on zero, and apply brakes if appropriate. If the scales are 'stand on' type ensure the patient stands on scales centrally, with feet slightly apart, and keeps still.	To ensure patient safety and promote accuracy of reading.
4. Perform steps 7-10 of the common steps (pp. 104-105).	To ensure that: • the patient is safe, comfortable and receiving the appropriate care; • the results have been documented in the patient's records; • the equipment is clean and in working order.

Evidence base: Dougherty and Lister (2011); RCN (2011b)

Assisting a patient to eat and drink

☑ What is normal
It is normal for patients, children included, to eat and drink with only minimal assistance, so remember to enable the patient to be as independent as possible.

☑ Before you start
Remember the common steps for all clinical measurements (pp. 104–105).

Check the patient's plan of care to ascertain whether there is a known swallowing difficulty.

☑ Essential equipment
Utensils – adapted if appropriate

Crockery and any necessary adapted items, such as a plate guard

Clothing protection for the patient, such as disposable covers or napkins, as required

The meal and a suitable drink

☑ Field-specific considerations
When caring for a patient with a learning disability, ascertaining their likes and dislikes is imperative to maintaining nutritional needs.

Many mental health conditions can affect appetite and the ability to prepare food as well as to eat and drink normally, so extra support may be required.

For children, age-appropriate food and choice of utensils are important safety issues.

Elderly patients may not eat or drink adequately due to problems with dentures and oral hygiene, plus the accessibility of food, or because of the effects of medication.

☑ Care-setting considerations
It is possible to assist a patient to eat and drink in any care setting. In community settings you may need to involve other agencies to help a patient maintain adequate nutrition throughout the whole day.

☑ What to watch out for and action to take
If the patient seems to have any difficulty swallowing at any time, stop immediately and report your concerns straight away to your mentor or another registered nurse.

When assisting a patient to eat or drink, you should also assess:

- the patient's positioning and ability to mobilize;
- their neurological condition – are they alert and responsive?
- any signs or complaints of pain or discomfort;
- the patient's or relative's views, as these may provide you with important additional information.

The information gained from these observations will enable you to fully assess the patient's condition, institute appropriate treatment as necessary and escalate needs care to senior nurses and the medical team.

Step	Reason and patient-centred care considerations
1. Perform steps 1-6 of the common steps (pp. 104-105).	To prepare the patient and yourself to undertake the skill.
2. Prepare the patient for the meal by: • Offering toilet and hand-washing facilities before the meal arrives. • Ascertain where the patient wishes to eat. • If using a bed table remove surplus equipment, particularly items such as sputum pots and vomit bowls. Clean the table and ensure it is at the correct height. • Collect the correct diet for the patient and the utensils they require. • Ensure you have a supply of fresh water or appropriate fluid.	To empower the patient and reduce infection risks. A social environment is often preferred to encourage normality, but some may wish to eat alone. To promote an environment conducive to eating and drinking. To ensure everything is to hand so you do not have to leave the patient.
3. Position yourself close to the patient, at the same level as them, in a comfortable position.	To promote the patient's dignity and ensure you are in a position that protects your back.
4. Ensure the patient approves of the food choice and that food is at an appropriate temperature and consistency.	To empower the patient and prevent harm from heat or swallowing difficulties.
5. Offer as much or as little assistance as is required. Whilst assisting the patient ensure pace is correct by asking for feedback. Ensure you offer food in the order the patient wishes, following their preferences. Communicate appropriately with the patient whilst they are eating, to make the experience a sociable and enjoyable one.	To empower the patient whilst promoting autonomy and dignity.

Step	Reason and patient-centred care considerations
6. Remember to offer and encourage fluids at frequent intervals whilst the patient is eating.	To aid swallowing and promote digestion.
7. Ensure the patient is not rushed and has sufficient time to complete their meal.	To ensure the patient eats and drinks the amount they wish.
8. Clear away crockery and utensils; offer patient appropriate hygiene, such as hand-washing, mouth care, clean dentures and clean bed table.	To promote patient comfort and a clean environment.
9. Leave patient in a comfortable, upright position for at least thirty minutes, with their call bell to hand.	To promote digestion and ensure patient safety. For children this will depend on their condition and stage of development, but in general aim to disturb the child as little as possible after feeding and encourage quiet activities for a while.
10. Perform steps 7-10 of the common steps (pp. 104-105).	

Evidence base: Dougherty and Lister (2011); NICE (2006, 2012b); RCN (2011b)

Passing a nasogastric tube

☑ **What is normal?**

Many patients who we care for will be able to maintain their own nutrition and fluids, however, some patients may need additional help. When this is necessary it is essential we follow the NICE (2012b) quality standards for nutritional support in adults. There are two ways we can provide nutrition for patients who can't swallow safely. A nasogastric tube can be passed or a gastrostomy created. There are advantages and disadvantages to both methods. A nasogastric tube is inserted quickly and easily, however, they need replacing frequently and patient acceptance is often poor (SIGN, 2012). If the tube is going to be used for feeding it is crucial the position of the tube is ascertained correctly to avoid inadvertent placement in the lungs, which if undetected, can have fatal consequences.

☑ Before you start
Remember the common steps for all care delivered to assist patients.

☑ Essential equipment
Clinically clean tray/receptacle
Fine bore naso-gastric tube – adult 6 FG – 10 FG / introducer
Syringe 50ml (catheter tip or luer slip to fit end of tube)
Disposable cup 3/4 full with tap water – to lubricate n/g tube
Cotton buds/tissue
Universal pH indicator paper/strips
Disposable gloves – non-sterile
Hypoallergenic adhesive tape
Denture bowl – where required
Disposable paper sheet
Glass of iced water **if not contraindicated**

☑ Field specific considerations
If assisting a patient who has a learning disability/any cognitive impairment or a child, it is important to ascertain their level of understanding. In these cases it may be appropriate to have parent(s) or carers present to help reassure the patient.

☑ Care setting considerations
Can be in any care setting: acute, rehabilitation, community hospital or home. NICE (2012b) sets out quality standards. These include standards for carers who manage nasogastric tubes.

☑ What to watch out for and action to take
Correct preparation and positioning of the patient can help you pass the nasogastric tube safely. If an obstruction is felt when introducing into the nose try the other nostril. Seek help from a colleague if in doubt. If a patient shows signs of distress: gasping or cyanosis stop the procedure immediately and remove the tube. Always check the position of the tube before use as displaced tubes can be fatal.

☑ Helpful Hints – Do I …?
- Gloves and aprons must be worn as contact with body fluid is anticipated.
- Hand hygiene must be performed before touching a patient, before clean/aseptic procedures, after body fluid exposure/risk, after touching a patient and after touching a patient's surroundings.
- Waste should be disposed of in a clinical waste bag if it is contaminated with blood/body fluids/excreta.

Step	Reason and patient-centred care considerations
1. Perform steps 1-6 of the common steps (pp. 104-105).	To prepare the patient and yourself to undertake the skill.
2. As you explain the procedure also arrange a signal by which a patient can tell you that they need you to stop (e.g. raising hand).	So patient feels they have some control – this should help to reduce anxiety.
3. Request/assist the patient to sit in a semi-upright position in the bed or chair. Support the patient's head with a pillow. The unconscious or dense hemiplegic patient should be placed flat in bed with one pillow under the head.	To allow for an easier passage of the tube. This position enables swallowing and ensures that the epiglottis is not obstructing the oesophagus.
4. Clean the patient's nostrils, if required. Encourage the patient to sniff with one nostril closed at a time.	This is to make the procedure more comfortable for the patient and removes any obstructions/ensures patency of the nasal cavity.
5. Request the patient to/or remove their dentures (if appropriate) and place in denture bowl.	This is so you do not displace dentures with the tube.
6. Protect the patient's clothing with a disposable paper sheet. To maintain patient dignity and comfort.	To minimize the risk of cross infection.
7. Wash and dry hands again.	To prevent cross infection.
8. Put on gloves.	To protect hands from body fluids.
9. Holding the n/g tube estimate the distance from the patient's ear lobe to the bridge of the nose and then to the lower end of the xiphisternum, without making contact with the skin or patient's clothing. Recent research (Taylor et al., 2014) indicates that the NEX (nose-ear-xiphisternum) measurement may not be long enough to reach the stomach, so they suggest adding 10cm but state	To provide an indication of the length of tube required to reach the patient's stomach.

Step	Reason and patient-centred care considerations
10. Follow manufacturer's instructions regarding visual checks and recommendations if using a guide wire.	To ensure safe effective use of the equipment.
11. Dip the tube in water (do not use lubricating gel as it gives an acid reaction) (Cunha et al., 2014).	To activate the external lubricant thus reducing friction between the mucous membrane and the tube.
12. Gently insert the tube through the nostril and slowly advance it along the nasal passage. If an obstruction is felt, withdraw slightly then advance the tube again at a slightly different angle. Gentle rotation of the tube can be helpful.	To facilitate passage of the tube by following the natural anatomy of the nose.
13. Request the patient to swallow as the tube is advanced. Sips of iced water may be offered to facilitate this **unless contraindicated.**	To facilitate closure of the epiglottis enabling the tube to pass into the oesophagus.
14. Continue to advance the tube until the length required has been passed. If an obstruction is felt do not force, withdraw the tube slightly and attempt to reinsert or withdraw completely and repass, or try another nostril.	To maintain patient safety.
15. Secure the tube to the cheek using hypoallergenic adhesive tape and hook over the ear.	To maintain the tube in position and keeping it out of the patient's visual field and avoiding friction to the nose/prevent allergic reaction. Change tape daily and use alternate sides of nose to prevent from becoming sore.
16. Confirm tube is in the stomach by withdrawing gastric content and checking on pH indicator paper/strips and/or perform a chest/upper abdominal X-ray. Please refer to your local policy for guidance.	To ensure the tube is correctly placed in the stomach - wrongly placed/or falsely verified tubes can be fatal.

Step	Reason and patient-centred care considerations
17. (a) Fill a syringe with 10ml of tap water and slowly flush the tube. (b) Gently remove the guide wire from the tube and discard. NOTE: Once the position has been confirmed remove the guide wire. To remove the guide wire attach an enteral dispenser (syringe) containing 10mls of water to the end of the tube and slowly inject the water down the tube. This activates the internal lubricant in the tube and aids removal. The tube should be held firmly at the tip of the nose to ensure that the tube stays in the position as the guide wire is removed. **The guide wire should never be reinserted while the tube is still in the patient.**	To facilitate the easy removal of the guide wire from the tube. Remember to always check the position of the tube **before** flushing as aspiration pneumonia can be caused if the tube is misplaced in the lungs and pH testing may be affected leading to a false positive reading (NPSA, 2012).
18. Measure all the visible tube from the tip of the nose and record in patient documentation.	To provide a record to help detect if the tube has moved (NPSA, 2011). Accurate record keeping promotes patient safety (NMC 2009).
19. Clean dentures if removed. Either replace or leave in bowl with clean water.	For patient oral hygiene and comfort.
20. Perform steps 7-10 of the common steps (pp. 104-105).	To ensure that the: • patient is safe, comfortable and receiving the appropriate care. • results have been documented in the patient's records. • any equipment is clean and ready to be reused.

Evidence Base: NICE (2012b); National Patient Safety Agency (2011, 2012); NMC (2009, 2015); SIGN (2012)

Confirmation of position of a nasogastric tube

☑ What is normal?
The position of a fine bore n/g tube should always be checked:

- After initial placement
- Before commencing feed
- Prior to administration of medicines if feed not in progress
- At least once daily if on continuous feeds
- After vomiting, excessive coughing, prolonged hiccoughing or oro-pharyngeal suction
- When there is any suggestion of tube displacement
- If there are any new or unexplained respiratory sounds

☑ What to watch out for and action to take
Following evidence based review in 2005 and 2011 by NPSA only two methods can confirm the gastric position of a N/G tube – the pH of the tube aspirate and X-ray, and that X-ray should only be a second line if no aspirate and pH reading is obtained. Check your local policy for guidance.

If a nasogastric tube is not tolerated, perhaps due to poor patient compliance, then discuss with multidisciplinary team and consider creation of a gastrostomy.

☑ Requirements
1. Clean tray
2. Syringe (50 ml)
3. **Universal pH indicator paper/strips** (only pH strips with a clear (**CE mark**) should be used (NPSA 2011))
4. Disposable gloves – non-sterile
5. N/G tube position confirmation record or N/G tube placement checklist if tube has been placed/replaced

Step	Reason and patient-centred care considerations
1. Perform steps 1-6 of the common steps (pp. 104-105).	To prepare the patient and yourself to undertake the skill.
Wash hands and put on gloves.	To minimize the risk of cross infection.

Step	Reason and patient-centred care considerations
2. Attach new clean 50 ml syringe to n/g tube and withdraw plunger to obtain gastric content. Detach syringe from n/g tube. If no aspirate obtained use these techniques recommended in the NPSA (2011) decision tree: ADULTS • If possible turn an adult onto left side • Inject 10-20 ml air through the tube and then gently withdraw plunger. Wait 15-30 minutes before aspirating again • Advance or withdraw tube by 20cm CHILDREN/INFANTS (not neonates) (NPSA 2011) • Inject 1-5 ml into the tube using a syringe • Wait for 15-30 minutes before aspirating again • Advance or withdraw tube by 1-2 cm ALL • Give mouth care to nil orally patients • Do not use water to flush until tube position confirmed	It is recognized that obtaining aspirate from fine bore tubes can be difficult. This stimulates gastric secretion of acid. To prevent harm to patient.
3. Put small amount of aspirate onto pH indicator paper/strip.	Follow manufacturer's guidelines for pH indicator strips to ensure accuracy of reading.
4. Compare indicator paper to colour and check pH acceptable to commence use of tube.	A pH of 1 to 5.5 indicates that the tube is positioned correctly and is safe to use. However if the reading has a pH of 5 to 6, then a second competent person should check the result and/or retest (O'Donnell, 2011).

Step	Reason and patient-centred care considerations
5. If unable to confirm position by aspirate then an X-ray will be necessary.	**A pH of 6 or above could indicate misplacement of the tube and should not be used** (NPSA 2011). To avoid false readings tubes MUST NOT be flushed with water prior to confirming position (NPSA, 2012).
6. The method of confirming position should always be documented with the pH obtained where appropriate.	Accurate record keeping promotes patient safety (NMC, 2009).
7. Perform steps 7-10 of the common steps (pp. 104-105).	To ensure that the: • patient is safe, comfortable and receiving the appropriate care. • results have been documented in the patients records. • any equipment is clean and ready to be reused.

Evidence Base: National Patient Safety Agency (2011, 2012); NMC (2009, 2015); SIGN (2012)

Maintaining a nasogastric tube

☑ **What is normal?**

NG tubes are prone to displacement and care is required to ensure they are retained in the correct positon. Skin condition should be monitored carefully as the tube and tape can cause sores.

☑ **Before you start**

Remember the common steps for all care delivered to assist patients.

☑ **Essential equipment**

Patient's toiletries
Bowl of water
Towel
Shaver (if required)
Tissues
Hypoallergenic Tape

Mouth wash
Vomit bowl (to rinse out mouth)

☑ Field specific considerations
If assisting a patient who has a learning disability/any cognitive impairment or a child, it is important to ascertain their level of understanding. In these cases it may be appropriate to have parent(s) or carers present to help reassure the patient.

☑ Care setting considerations
Can be in any care setting: acute, rehabilitation, community hospital or home.

☑ What to watch out for and action to take
Red sore areas around ears and nose. Change tape and positon of tube regularly.

☑ Helpful Hints – Do I …?
- Gloves and aprons must be worn as contact with body fluid is anticipated.
- Hand hygiene must be performed before touching a patient, before clean/aseptic procedures, after body fluid exposure/risk, after touching a patient and after touching a patient's surroundings.
- Waste should be disposed of in a clinical waste bag if it is contaminated with blood/body fluids/excreta.

Step	Reason and patient centred care considerations
Nasal Hygiene: Gently clean area. Encourage patient to blow nose if necessary. Change position of tube exit site ensuring tape not pulling tube too tightly.	To allow nostrils to remain unblocked. To prevent pressure sore.
Oral Hygiene: Regular oral hygiene with mouth washes. Encourage patient to brush teeth and gums regularly.	Patient often breathes with n/g tube insitu so the mouth can become dry. If patient on nil by mouth then saliva may not be produced as normal.
Facial Cleansing: Daily removal of tape and normal face washing. Avoid use of moisturizer where tape is to be applied.	Area around tube often neglected for fear of disturbing tube. Excess oils can make it difficult to secure tape.

Step	Reason and patient centred care considerations
Shaving as normal for men.	Promote patient-centred care.
Changing tape: Carefully remove all old tape before applying new. Skin condition below tape should be checked	Tape can lose its adherence qualities. Prevent damage to skin.
Flushing for maintenance: Tube should be flushed before and after use.	To ensure that tube remains patent.

Evidence base: Dougherty and Lister (2011)

Removing a nasogastric tube

☑ **What is normal?**
It is normal to replace naso gastric tubes every 10-28 days depending on the type of tube and material it is made from; always follow the manufacturers guidelines (SIGN, 2013).

☑ **Before you start**
Remember the common steps for all care delivered to assist patients.

☑ **Essential equipment**
Clean tray
Tissues
Disposable gloves – non-sterile
Disposable paper sheet
Polythene bag

☑ **Field specific considerations**
If assisting a patient who has a learning disability/any cognitive impairment or a child, it is important to ascertain their level of understanding. In these cases it may be appropriate to have parent(s) or carers present to help reassure the patient.

☑ **Care setting considerations**
Can be in any care setting: acute, rehabilitation, community hospital or home.

☑ **Helpful Hints – Do I ...?**

- Gloves and aprons must be worn if contact with blood/body fluids/excreta is anticipated or the patient is in isolation.
- Hand hygiene must be performed before touching a patient, before clean/aseptic procedures, after body fluid exposure/risk, after touching a patient and after touching a patient's surroundings.
- Waste should be disposed of in a clinical waste bag if it is contaminated with blood/body fluids/excreta

Step	Reason and patient-centred care considerations
1. Perform steps 1-6 of the common steps (pp. 104-105).	To prepare the patient and yourself to undertake the skill.
Wash hands and put on gloves.	To minimize the risk of cross infection.
2. Protect patient's clothing with a disposable paper sheet.	To promote patient dignity and protect clothing.
3. Remove tape securing tube. If nasal bridle is in situ please cut tape above clip.	To allow tube to move freely.
4. Pinch tube and gently withdraw tube into polythene bag.	To prevent spillage on removal through oesophagus.
5. Give patient tissue to clean nasal area/blow nose.	Promote patient comfort and dignity.
6. Perform steps 7-10 of the common steps (pp. 104-105).	To ensure that the: • patient is safe, comfortable and receiving the appropriate care. • results have been documented in the patient's records. • any equipment is clean and ready to be reused.

Evidence-base: NMC (2009); SIGN (2012)

Caring for a PEG (pertcutaneous endoscopic gastrostomy)*

*This skill relates to patients who have a well established PEG tube site.

☑ What is normal?

Healthy individuals consume food and fluids by eating and drinking. Food and fluids are taken orally and begin the process of digestion in the mouth. Some patients are required to receive fluid and nutrition via a PEG tube, an example being someone who has had a stroke and can no longer swallow. PEG tube sites should be cleaned daily. Some patients may be self-caring and will do this whilst showering or bathing.

☑ Before you start

Remember the common steps for all care delivered to assist patients.

☑ Essential equipment

Suitable personal protective equipment (PPE), in this case, gloves and apron are sufficient
Bactericidal alcohol hand gel
Soap and warm water
Gauze swabs and/or cotton buds
Towel (or something to dry the skin)
Dressings (if applicable)

☑ Field specific considerations

If assisting a patient who has a learning disability, it is important to ascertain their level of understanding.

As is appropriate depending upon the age of a child, encourage and assist parents or carers to become involved in care to maintain as far as is possible their normal caring role.

☑ Care setting considerations

PEG tube care may occur in any care setting.

☑ What to watch out for and action to take

This procedure could be considered to be intimate and may cause the patient embarrassment or distress. Ensure you promote the patient's dignity and provide privacy at all times.

☑ Helpful Hints – Do I …?

- Gloves and aprons must be worn if contact with blood/body fluids/excreta is anticipated or the patient is in isolation.
- Hand hygiene must be performed before touching a patient, before clean/aseptic procedures, after body fluid exposure/risk, after touching a patient and after touching a patient's surroundings.
- Waste should be disposed of in a clinical waste bag if it is contaminated with blood/body fluids/excreta.

Step	Reason and patient-centred care considerations
1. Perform steps 1-6 of the common steps (pp. 104-105).	To prepare the patient and yourself to undertake the skill.
2. Position the patient for the procedure.	To allow ease of access, maintain patient comfort and to adhere to moving and handling regulations.
3. Remove any dressings which may be in-situ.	To allow inspection of the PEG Tube site.
4. Examine the skin around the PEG tube looking for: • Redness/inflammation/ swelling/foul smelling odour • Discharge • Encrustation • Excess skin tissue development	To assess for signs of infection, leakage from the site or granulation tissue (a recognized minor complication). If any of these are present, seek advice from your mentor or other registered nurse/ healthcare professional.
5. Clean the site with warm soap and water, using swabs/cotton buds to gently remove any encrustation which may have developed.	To cleanse the skin.
6. Rinse the area.	To remove any soap/residue which may cause skin irritation. Powders or creams should be avoided as this may cause skin irritation.
7. Dry the area thoroughly, using cotton buds to dry under the PEG tube.	To prevent any deterioration of the skin.
8. Apply any prescribed creams/ ointments.	For therapeutic effect.
9. Apply dressing if required.	To protect the PEG tube site. Dressings should only be needed if there is continued discharge.
10. Perform steps 7-10 of the common steps (pp. 104-105).	To ensure that the: • patient is safe, comfortable and receiving the appropriate care. • results have been documented in the patient's records. • Any equipment is clean and ready to be reused.

Evidence base: Simons and Remington (2013)

Stoma care

☑ **Essential Equipment**

Suitable appliance (stoma pouch or bag), scissors, measuring guide, gloves and apron, access to sink or bowl of warm water, wipes, measuring jug if required, receptacle for soiled disposable items.

Appliances come as a one piece closed system, one piece drainable system or a two piece system.

☑ **Care setting considerations**

Always ensure you have the equipment required to safely meet the patient's needs in your current setting. For example, in a community setting it may be necessary to dispose of waste in the rubbish bin. This should be double bagged first.

The size of the appliance is determined by measuring the stoma using the measuring device that accompanies the appliances. Some appliances need to be cut to size. Too large an opening in the bag exposes the skin to the bag contents and too small an opening may cause trauma to the stoma.

☑ **What to watch out for/action to take**

Whilst maintaining stoma care:

- the colour of the stoma and surrounding skin
- the consistency of the faeces
- any complaints of pain or discomfort

The information gained from these observations will enable you to fully assess the condition of the patient's skin and if necessary plan any changes in treatment plus evaluate whether the current treatment is effective. Any abnormalities or changes must be reported to a relevant individual and recorded in the patient's notes.

☑ **Field specific considerations**

Learning Disability – it may be important to ascertain what a patient's usual routine is, as they may not be able to tell you. Assisting a patient to develop their ability to maintain their elimination needs can be an important step towards independence.

Mental Health – patients who are severely depressed may not view stoma care as important, so both physical and psychological support could be required.

Child – encourage and assist parents or carers to be involved to maintain the usual routine. Supporting, educating and enabling parents or carers to adopt new care practices within any environment is an important nursing role.

Step	Reason and patient-centred care considerations
1. The first step of any procedure is to introduce yourself to the patient, explain the procedure and gain their consent.	There will be differences in how you go about this for children or those with mental health or learning disabilities as not all patients will be able to provide consent, but they will be able to assent. It could be that the procedure is one normally undertaken by the patient's family or carer, or they may express the wish to be involved in the care you are about to deliver. If this is so, and it is appropriate, it is an opportunity to maintain the patient's usual routine, or you could support the patient's family or carer in adapting their usual routine to meet the patient's changed care needs.
2. Gather the equipment required. Ensure these are clean as appropriate.	To ensure you are ready to complete the procedure.
3. Ensure privacy, so close doors and curtains/blinds as necessary. If you are at a patient's bed-space ensure you draw the curtains fully.	Patients will need to feel comfortable when carrying out stoma care. Maintains privacy, dignity and comfort. Caring for a patient's hygiene is a personal and intimate procedure which takes time to perform with dignity.
4. Ensure the patient is in a comfortable position, adjust clothing to expose the abdomen.	To ensure the area is visible for the patient to access or to observe.
5. Wash your hands, put on an apron and gloves.	To prevent contamination from body fluids.
6. As appropriate encourage the patient to undertake as much of the process as possible.	Promotes independence.
7. Place disposable wipes around stoma site.	To protect surrounding skin from spills or leakage.
8. Empty the appliance and if necessary measure contents.	To monitor output and to ensure easier removal.

Step		Reason and patient-centred care considerations
9.	Remove appliance and dispose of in a disposable bag or receptacle.	To ensure safe disposal.
10.	Wash skin surrounding the stoma with warm water and wipes.	To remove excess faeces and ensure skin is intact.
11.	Observe surrounding skin for signs of redness and excoriation and also colour and condition of stoma.	To ensure complications are identified promptly.
12.	Dry skin thoroughly around stoma site and apply barrier wipes or sprays.	To prevent excoriation and to ensure the new appliance will be securely attached.
13.	Prepare appliance and place in position.	Ensure appliance is prepared as per manufacturers guidelines. This will ensure skin is protected.
14.	Dispose of any waste products as per guidelines.	To ensure safe disposal.
15.	Remove your apron and perform hand hygiene and document in the patient's notes the care you have given and any relevant observations of pressure areas etc.	Reduces the risk of infection. Maintains patient safety and accurate records.
16.	Offer or support the patient and ensure the patient is comfortable.	

Evidence base: Baillie L. (2009); Doughtery and Lister (2011); NMC (2007, 2015)

Peripheral vascular cannula care

☑ **What is normal?**

Many patients who are cared for in an in-patient environment such as an acute hospital will have an intravenous peripheral cannula inserted. This device is usually located in the back of the hand or forearm but occasionally may be sited in other places such as the foot. It is used to provide intravenous medications and/or fluids. Blood samples may be obtained at the time of insertion but that should not be the only reason for inserting a cannula. Cannulas should be removed if no longer required.

☑ Before you start
Remember the common steps for all care delivered to assist patients. This procedure uses the aseptic non-touch technique; make sure you are familiar with it.

☑ Essential equipment
Suitable personal protective equipment (PPE), in this case, gloves and apron are sufficient
Bactericidal alcohol hand gel
A clean trolley or surface for your equipment
Sterile dressing pack (containing sterile swabs) and normal saline
Antiseptic solution (as per local policy)
Transparent dressing (as per local policy)
Sharps bin (may be required)

☑ Field specific considerations
If assisting a patient who has a learning disability, it is important to ascertain their level of understanding.

As is appropriate depending upon the age of a child, encourage and assist parents or carers to become involved in care to maintain as far as is possible their normal caring role.

Reassurance may be required as some patients may associate peripheral vascular cannula care with the pain/discomfort of having the cannula inserted in the first place.

☑ Care setting considerations
Predominantly in an in-patient care setting.

☑ What to watch out for and action to take
Infection is a risk when patients have a peripheral vascular cannula in-situ; be aware of what the common signs and symptoms of infection are and report anything abnormal to your mentor or other registered healthcare professional.

☑ **Helpful Hints – Do I …?**

- Gloves and aprons must be worn if contact with blood/body fluids/excreta is anticipated or the patient is in isolation.
- Hand hygiene must be performed before touching a patient, before clean/aseptic procedures, after body fluid exposure/risk, after touching a patient and after touching a patient's surroundings.
- Waste should be disposed of in a clinical waste bag if it is contaminated with blood/body fluids/excreta.

Step	Reason and patient-centred care considerations
1. Perform steps 1-6 of the common steps (pp. 104-105).	To prepare the patient and yourself to undertake the skill.
2. Position the patient for the procedure.	To allow ease of access, maintain patient comfort and to adhere to moving and handling regulations.
3. Remove any dressings which may be in-situ.	To allow inspection of the cannula site.
4. Examine the skin around the cannula looking for: Redness/inflammation/swelling Discharge/bleeding	To assess for signs of infection. If any of these are present, seek advice from your mentor or other registered nurse/healthcare professional.
5. Clean the site with sterile swabs and normal saline, being careful not to dislodge the cannula.	To cleanse the skin and remove any residue which may cause skin irritation.
6. Dry the area thoroughly.	To prevent any deterioration of the skin.
7. Scrub the port(s) of the cannula using an antiseptic solution containing 70% isopropyl alcohol for 15 seconds or more (or as per local policy).	To remove any microbial contamination and reduce the risk of infection.

Step	Reason and patient-centred care considerations
8. Apply sterile, transparent dressing (as per local policy).	To allow visual inspection of the cannula site and reduce the risk of mechanical phlebitis. Do not secure with a bandage as this prevents the site from being observed.
9. Perform steps 7-10 of the common steps (pp. 104-105).	To ensure that the: • patient is safe, comfortable and receiving the appropriate care. • results have been documented in the patients records. • any equipment is clean and ready to be reused.

Evidence base: Dougherty and Lister (2011); Health Protection Scotland (2012); McCallum and Higgins (2012); NMC (2015)

ASSISTING PATIENTS WITH THEIR ELIMINATION NEEDS

MAIREAD COLLIE, DAVID J. HUNTER AND VALERIE FOLEY

Common steps for all elimination-related skills

☑ **Essential equipment – depends upon skill but is likely to include one or more of the following**

Suitable personal protective equipment (PPE)

Bedpan and paper cover, urinal, commode

Toilet paper

Equipment to enable the patient to wash their hands

Manual handling equipment and possibly assistance from another member of the healthcare team

Soap and warm water, single-use washcloths and towels

Sterile jug or container

Alcohol swabs

☑ **Field-specific considerations**

When caring for a patient with a learning disability it is important to know their level of understanding so that consent for and cooperation with the care can be gained. You will need to allow time to explain why you are doing the measurements and whether they will cause discomfort or pain.

Patients who have mental health problems may not understand the relevance of the care you plan to deliver. They may therefore withhold consent and you may need to refer to the Mental Capacity Act 2005 and best interest.

When assisting children with elimination needs, if possible it is usually helpful to have the parents or carers present to assist.

☑ **Care-setting considerations**

Assisting patients with elimination needs can occur within all settings, although you may not have all the equipment available to assist you. For example, in a patient's home you may not have manual handling equipment, so to ensure patient safety and your own, thorough risk assessments need to be undertaken.

☑ **What to watch out for and action to take**

Whilst assisting a patient with their elimination needs, as appropriate, you should also observe and assess:

- the condition of their skin;
- their ability to move or mobilize independently;
- their neurological condition – are they alert and responsive?;
- any signs or complaints of pain or discomfort;
- the patient's or relatives' views – for example, saying that their needs have changed or that they are experiencing problems.

The information gained from these observations will enable you to fully assess the patient's condition and institute appropriate treatment as necessary.

☑ **Helpful hints – Do I …?**

- Gloves and aprons must be worn if contact with blood/body fluids/excreta is anticipated or the patient is in isolation.
- Hand hygiene must be performed before touching a patient, before clean/aseptic procedures, after body fluid exposure/risk, after touching a patient and after touching a patient's surroundings.
- Waste should be disposed of in a clinical waste bag if it is contaminated with blood/body fluids/excreta.

Step	Reason and patient-centred care considerations
1. The first step of any procedure is to introduce yourself to the patient, explain the procedure and gain their consent.	Fully informed consent may not always be possible if the patient is a child or has mental health problems or learning disabilities, but even in these circumstances, every effort should be made to explain the procedure in terms that the patient can understand. This is not only respectful of their individual human rights, but also helps to ensure that they will be more accepting of the treatment and that their anxieties are reduced.

Step	Reason and patient-centred care considerations
	For patients who are unable to provide consent because they are unconscious, advice should be sought from your mentor or another qualified nurse.
2. Gather the equipment required (see individual skills for equipment required). Ensure these are clean as appropriate and in working order.	Ensures the skill is performed effectively. Reduces the chance of infection and maintains patient and nurse safety.
3. Clear sufficient space within the environment, for example around the bed space or chair.	Enables clear access for the patient and the nurse to safely use the equipment required.
4. Wash your hands with soap and water before you start any care activity. Apron and gloves should only be worn if appropriate.	Wearing an apron and gloves as part of personal protective equipment (PPE) is a standard infection-control procedure when dealing with body fluids or patients in isolation. Ensure your use of PPE such as gloves and disposable aprons is appropriate by considering the individual patient situation and the risk presented.
5. Ensure you promote patient dignity and privacy as appropriate, for example by drawing curtains or moving the patient to a bathroom if at all possible.	Elimination needs are intimate and personal. At all times you need to maintain patient privacy, dignity and comfort as required.
6. Patients need to be in a comfortable position.	To promote patient comfort and reduce anxiety.
7. After performing the skill ensure the patient is in a comfortable position, with drinks and call bells available as necessary.	Promotes patient comfort and ensures they are well nourished and hydrated.
8. Discard PPE, any single-use equipment and other used materials as per policy. Clean any equipment used as per the relevant policy every time it is used and perform hand hygiene.	To prevent cross-infection and maintain equipment in working condition.

Step	Reason and patient-centred care considerations
9. Document findings as appropriate, for example on the patient's observation chart and/or in the patient's notes.	Maintains patient safety and accurate records.
10. If any abnormalities are observed, escalate to senior nursing staff or your mentor immediately.	It is vital to report any abnormalities to a registered nurse immediately so they can ensure the patient receives the care required.

Evidence base: NMC (2009, 2015); WHO (2009)

Assessing bowel function

☑ **What is normal?**
'Normal' bowel function can vary greatly: some patients open their bowels daily, others every two or three days. If possible it is best to ask the patient what is 'normal' for them and whether they take laxatives.

☑ **Before you start**
Remember the common steps for all care delivered to assist patients with their elimination needs (pp. 130–132).

Other factors need to be considered when assessing a patient's bowel function, as this will enable you to assess the patient's overall condition. As you approach the patient observe them carefully to assess whether they are well nourished and hydrated. Do they look in good health or do they appear unwell, and are they able to move unaided?

☑ **Essential equipment**
Relevant documentation with regard to bowel assessment. This can vary between patients depending upon the field, as well as between care settings. Appropriate personal protective equipment (PPE).

☑ **Field-specific considerations**
If assessing a patient who has a learning disability, it is important to ascertain their level of understanding. If appropriate, involve a family member or carer in the discussion.

When assessing a patient with mental health problems their level of capacity may need to be considered, so they may require support and assistance to enable them to recognize that they are constipated.

As appropriate depending upon the age of a child, encourage and assist their parents or carers to become involved, as they will provide useful information.

☑ **Care-setting considerations**

An assessment of bowel function can be undertaken in any care setting.

☑ **What to watch out for and action to take**

Remember that the questions you are going to ask may cause anxiety and embarrassment.

If any abnormalities are found this must be reported to a qualified nurse immediately and recorded in the patient's notes.

Step	Reason and patient-centred care considerations
1. Perform steps 1-6 of the common steps (pp. 130-132).	To prepare the patient and yourself to undertake the skill.
2. Document the history of the present bowel complaint.	To gain an understanding of the patient's needs and to direct management or treatment decisions.
3. Undertake a holistic assessment of the patient's condition, which includes details of their diet, fluids, mobility, dexterity, cognitive function and usual environment.	To obtain a comprehensive and holistic assessment which may identify the underlying reason for the patient's altered bowel habit, whether constipation or diarrhoea.
4. Document the patient's usual bowel pattern.	To ascertain what is 'normal' for the patient.
5. Ask the patient what medications they are currently taking.	To assess if medication has affected the normal bowel routine.
6. Ask the patient to identify their stool formation using the Bristol Stool Chart.	Enables clear identification of the patient's needs and allows effective management.

Step	Reason and patient-centred care considerations
7. As is appropriate within the care setting, ensure that future bowel actions are monitored and accurately recorded.	To monitor condition and detect abnormalities.
8. Develop a plan of care in partnership with the patient and their parents or carers as appropriate.	To produce a clear plan of care to be delivered to the patient and ensure that the patient is aware of and happy with the ongoing management of the condition.
9. Perform steps 7-10 of the common steps (pp. 130-132).	To ensure that: • the patient is safe, comfortable and receiving the appropriate care; • the results have been documented in the patient's records.

Evidence base: NMC (2009, 2015)

Assisting a patient to use a bedpan, urinal or commode

☑ **What is normal?**
Female patients may need to use a bedpan or commode to both micturate and defecate; male patients may prefer to micturate in a urinal, which may be easier if they stand up (if this is appropriate).

☑ **Before you start**
Remember the common steps for all care delivered to assist patients with their elimination needs (pp. 130–132).

☑ **Essential equipment**
Appropriate personal protective equipment (PPE)
Appropriate bedpan and paper cover or commode or urinal and paper cover
Toilet paper
Facilities to allow the patient to wash their hands
Manual handling equipment as required
Possible assistance from a further member of the healthcare team

Step	Reason and patient-centred care considerations
1. Perform steps 1-6 of the common steps (pp. 130-132).	To prepare the patient and yourself to undertake the skill.
Commode	
2. Assess the moving and handling needs of the patient. Ensure the patient's weight does not exceed the manufacturer's recommendations.	To maintain a safe environment and to determine whether or not additional assistance is required.
3. Take the equipment to the bedside, checking that the wheels on the commode are secured and that there is a bedpan receiver placed under the commode.	A comfortable position may make it easier for the patient to open their bowels.
Remove the commode cover and assist the patient to transfer from bed/chair to the commode. Ensure the patient is comfortable.	To ensure patient safety.
4. Check the patient is positioned correctly on the commode.	Checking the position will reduce the risk of spillage and associated contamination or cross-infection.
Bedpan or urinal	
2. Assess the moving and handling needs of the patient.	
3. Remove the bedclothes and, if the patient is able, assist them to sit upright. Ask the patient (or use moving and handling equipment if required) to raise their hips/buttocks to allow the bedpan or urinal to be correctly positioned. If the patient cannot raise their hips/buttocks, a rolling motion may be used with appropriate moving and handling techniques to roll the patient onto the bedpan. Support with pillow if required.	
4. When the patient is on the bedpan or has the urinal in position, ask them to move their legs slightly apart so that you can check the position is correct.	

Step	Reason and patient-centred care considerations
5. If safe to do so, leave the patient, ensuring that toilet paper is close at hand and giving them a nurse call button. Cover the patient's legs with a towel or sheet. This step is not possible if you are supporting a patient to use a urinal whilst standing.	To maintain privacy and dignity.
6. When the patient has finished using the bedpan, commode or urinal, you may need to assist them with personal hygiene. As indicated, select the appropriate PPE and clean the patient's bottom using toilet paper, wiping from front to back. Skin cleanser or warm soapy water may be required.	Assisting the patient to be clean will ensure patient comfort. Wiping from front to back will reduce the spread of infection from the bowel to the urethra (especially in women).
7. Pat the skin dry after assisting the patient with their personal hygiene.	To prevent deterioration of the patient's skin.
8. Help the patient to wash and dry their hands.	To promote patient comfort, dignity and infection control.
9. Perform steps 7–10 of the common steps (pp. 130–132).	To ensure that: • the patient is safe, comfortable and receiving the appropriate care. • the results have been documented in the patient's records. • any equipment is clean and ready to be reused.

Evidence base: Ballentyne and Ness (2009); NMC (2009, 2015); Oxford University Hospitals NHS Trust (2013)

☑ **Field-specific considerations**

If assisting a patient who has a learning disability or cognitive impairment, it is important to ascertain their level of understanding.

As appropriate depending upon the age of a child, encourage and assist parents or carers to become involved in care to maintain their normal caring role as far as is possible.

☑ **Care-setting considerations**

A patient can be assisted to use a bedpan, commode or urinal in any care setting.

☑ **What to watch out for and action to take**

Elimination is an intimate and personal activity. Ensure you promote the patient's dignity and provide privacy at all times.

Performing catheter care

☑ **What is normal?**

Catheter care should be undertaken as a part of the patient's routine hygiene care.

☑ **Before you start**

Remember the common steps for all care delivered to assist patients with their elimination needs (pp. 130–132).

☑ **Essential equipment**

Appropriate personal protective equipment (PPE)
Soap and warm water
Single-use washcloths
Towel

☑ **Field-specific considerations**

If assisting a patient who has a learning disability, it is important to ascertain their level of understanding.

As appropriate depending upon the age of a child, encourage and assist parents or carers to become involved in care to maintain their normal caring role as far as is possible.

☑ **Care-setting considerations**

Catheter care can be undertaken in any care setting.

☑ **What to watch out for and action to take:**

Performing catheter care is an intimate and personal activity. Ensure you promote the patient's dignity and provide privacy at all times.

Step	Reason and patient-centred care considerations
1. Perform steps 1-6 of the common steps (pp. 130-132).	To prepare the patient and yourself to undertake the skill.
2. Assist the patient to be correctly positioned for the procedure.	To allow ease of access, maintain patient comfort and adhere to moving and handling regulations.
3. Clean the genital area using soap and water.	Soap and water are appropriate; anti-bacterial or antiseptic solutions are not required.
4. Perform meatal cleansing: a. in male patients by pulling back the foreskin (if uncircumcised). Note that the foreskin should not be forcibly pulled back. It can take untill the late teenage years before the foreskin can be retracted. Clean around the glans, moving away from the meatal opening; clean the area where the catheter enters the penis and then downwards along the catheter. Rinse and dry the area. Return the foreskin to the original position.	To reduce the risk of spreading infection. To expose the glans penis and the urethral meatus. To reduce contamination. To remove any buildup of smegma. To reduce the risk of irritation from soap and to maintain skin integrity. To reduce the risk of paraphimosis developing.
b. in female patients by gently parting the labia. Clean the area where the catheter enters the meatus and then downwards along the catheter. Rinse and dry the area.	To expose the inner genitals (labia minora) and the urethral meatus. To reduce contamination, particularly from the anus. To reduce the risk of irritation from soap and to maintain skin integrity.
5. Make sure that the area is completely dry.	To reduce the risk of skin breakdown. Talcum powder should be avoided as irritation may be caused.

Step	Reason and patient-centred care considerations
6. Ensure that the patient is comfortable and re-dressed following the procedure.	To promote patient comfort and dignity.
7. Perform steps 7-10 of the common steps (pp. 130-132).	To ensure that: • the patient is safe, comfortable and receiving the appropriate care; • the results have been documented in the patient's records; • any equipment is clean and ready to be reused.

Evidence base: Hunter (2012); Leaver (2007); NICE (2003); NMC (2015)

Emptying a patient's catheter bag

☑ What is normal?
Catheter bags should only be emptied when they are full, as each time you perform this procedure you are potentially introducing an infection risk.

☑ Before you start
Remember the common steps for all care delivered to assist patients with their elimination needs (pp. 130–132).

Do not forget that a catheter bag is attached to a patient and that you need to ask for their consent to perform this procedure.

☑ Essential equipment
Appropriate personal protective equipment (PPE)
Alcohol swabs
Sterile jug

☑ Field-specific considerations
If assisting a patient who has a learning disability, it is important to ascertain their level of understanding.

As appropriate depending upon the age of a child, encourage and assist parents or carers to become involved in care to maintain their normal caring role as far as is possible.

☑ **Care-setting considerations**

Emptying a catheter bag can be undertaken in any care setting.

☑ **What to watch out for and action to take**

Emptying a catheter bag can be seen by patients to be the same activity as using the toilet. Ensure you promote the patient's dignity and provide privacy at all times. If the patient's urine output is not being monitored frequently and you notice when emptying the bag that the patient has passed little or no urine, check the patient's fluid balance chart, as their catheter bag may have just been emptied. If this is not the case, you must inform your mentor or a registered nurse, as it may indicate a problem relating to catheter drainage or an alteration in the patient's condition.

Step	Reason and patient-centred care considerations
1. Perform steps 1–6 of the common steps (pp. 130–132).	To prepare the patient and yourself to undertake the skill.
2. Clean the outlet port of the catheter bag with the alcohol swab and allow to fully dry.	To reduce the risk of infection.
3. Open the port and allow the urine to drain into the jug.	To empty the bag and, if required, to allow measurement of the volume of urine passed.
4. Close the port and clean again with an alcohol swab.	To reduce the risk of infection.
5. Reposition the catheter bag and check that the patient is comfortable.	To ensure the patient is comfortable.
6. Cover the jug and transfer to the sluice where the urine can be disposed of. If required, the urine should be measured.	Reduce the risk of contamination. To monitor the patient's condition and to maintain accurate documentation.
7. Perform steps 7–10 of the common steps (pp. 130–132).	To ensure that: • the patient is safe, comfortable and receiving the appropriate care. • the results have been documented in the patient's records. • any equipment is clean and ready to be reused.

Evidence base: NHS Greater Glasgow and Clyde (2012); NMC (2015)

Urinalysis

☑ **Before you start**

Remember the common steps for all care delivered to assist patients with their elimination needs (pp. 130–132).

Assess the colour and smell of the urine.

☑ **Essential equipment**

White-top sterile specimen containers or bedpans are the most commonly used receptacles. To undertake accurate urinalysis the receptacle needs to be clean but not necessarily sterile, so any clean receptacle which can hold water may be used.

☑ **Care-setting considerations**

Can be measured in any care setting.

Ensure that the patient has the mobility necessary to use the commode, urinal or bedpan. If this is not the case offer assistance and support and apply safe patient moving techniques. Catheterization may be considered, but the need for this would be carefully risk-assessed.

Step	Reason and patient-centred care considerations
1. Perform steps 1-5 of the common steps (pp. 130-132).	To prepare the patient and yourself to undertake the skill.
2. Ensure the container you are going to use to obtain the specimen is appropriately labelled with the patient's identification details.	To ensure that you test the correct specimen.
3. First voided morning urine is best suited for urinalysis.	Its concentration provides the most reliable results.
4. It is best to test specimens immediately; if not possible then do so within two hours.	This provides the most reliable results.
5. After shaking the sample, briefly completely immerse the whole section of the strip where the test pads are located into freshly voided urine.	Shake the sample to ensure it is mixed so the concentration will be constant throughout. Dip the strip briefly to avoid dissolving out reagents from the test pads which would produce incorrect results.

Step	Reason and patient-centred care considerations
6. As you remove the strip from the sample, run its edge against the edge of the receptacle – apply the 'dip and drag' stages of the 'dip, drag, blot, read' technique.	To remove excess urine and prevent the strip from dripping.
7. Hold the strip horizontally.	To avoid potential mixing of reagents due to them running down the strip. This would cause cross-reactions that will produce unreliable results.
8. Remove excess urine by applying the 'blot' stage of the 'dip, drag, blot, read' technique. Blot the edge of the strip on absorbent material such as a paper towel. Take care not to touch the test pads and maintain the strip in a horizontal position.	To prevent the strip from dripping.
9. Compare all test pads with the corresponding colour chart. At the time specified, record all results. This is the 'read' stage of the 'dip, drag, blot, read' technique. Make sure that when you are comparing the test pads with the corresponding colour you do not hold the strip directly against the container, as there may be urine remaining on the strip which you would transfer to the container.	It is important to follow the timings specified to ensure that your results are correct. Colour changes that have occurred after two minutes are invalid and will not provide accurate results.
10. Perform steps 8-10 of the common steps (pp. 130-132).	To ensure that: • the patient is safe, comfortable and receiving the appropriate care; • the results have been documented in the patient's records.

Evidence base: Smith and Roberts (2011)

ASSISTING PATIENTS WITH THEIR HYGIENE NEEDS

CATHERINE DELVES-YATES

Common steps for all hygiene procedures

☑ **Essential equipment – depends upon skill but is likely to include one or more of the following**

Single-use bowls, warm water, towels, soap, incontinence pads, disposable washcloths, skin moisturizer or talc (if the patient wishes), clean clothes, nightwear or gown for the patient, clean bedlinen.

☑ **Field-specific considerations**

When assisting a patient with a learning disability it may be important to ascertain what a patient's usual hygiene routine is, as they may not be able to tell you. Assisting a patient to develop their ability to maintain their hygiene needs can be an important step towards independence.

Patients with mental health problems – who are severely depressed, for example – may not view their personal hygiene as important, so both physical and psychological support could be required. Those with a cognitive impairment such as dementia or psychosis may not realize or even understand what is needed.

When caring for a child, encourage and assist parents or carers to be involved in hygiene care to maintain the usual routine. Supporting, educating and enabling parents or carers to continue their care within any environment is an important nursing role.

☑ **Care-setting considerations**

It is not always possible to have all the equipment available to assist a patient to safely meet their hygiene needs in the exact manner they wish. For example, in a patient's home you may not have a hoist, so it may not be safe for them to use their bath; however, you can still assist them to meet their hygiene needs in a different way.

Always ensure you have the equipment required to safely meet the patient's needs in your current setting.

☑ What to watch out for/action to take

Whilst maintaining a patient's hygiene you should assess:

- the colour of the skin, lips, nail beds and sclera of their eyes;
- the location and appearance of any rashes;
- whether the skin is dry and/or flaky;
- the condition of pressure areas, for any bruises, open areas, pale or reddened areas; the appearance of any wounds and whether or not they are draining;
- any complaints of pain or discomfort;
- the temperature of the patient's skin.

The information gained from these observations will enable you to fully assess the condition of the patient's skin and if necessary plan any changes in treatment, plus evaluate whether the current treatment is effective.

☑ Helpful hints – Do I …?

- Gloves and aprons must be worn if contact with blood/body fluids/excreta is anticipated or the patient is in isolation.
- Hand hygiene must be performed before touching a patient, before clean/aseptic procedures, after body fluid exposure/risk, after touching a patient and after touching a patient's surroundings.
- Waste should be disposed of in a clinical waste bag if it is contaminated with blood/body fluids/excreta.
- Equipment must be cleaned as identified by the relevant policy every time it is used.

Step	Reason and patient-centred care considerations
1. The first step of any procedure is to introduce yourself to the patient, explain the procedure and gain their consent.	Fully informed consent may not always be possible if the patient is a child or has mental health problems or learning disabilities, but even in these circumstances, every effort should be made to explain the procedure in terms that the patient can understand. This is not only respectful of their individual human rights, but also helps to ensure

Step	Reason and patient-centred care considerations
	they will be more accepting of the treatment and that their anxieties are reduced.
	For patients who are unable to provide consent because they are unconscious, advice should be sought from your mentor or another qualified nurse.
	It could be that the procedure is one normally undertaken by the patient's family or carer, or they may express the wish to be involved in the care you are about to deliver. If this is so, and if it is appropriate, it is an opportunity to maintain the patient's usual routine, or you could support the patient's family or carer in adapting their usual routine to meet the patient's changed care needs.
2. Gather the equipment required (see relevant skill for details). Ensure these are clean as appropriate.	Reduces the chance of infection and maintains patient and nurse safety.
3. Clear sufficient space within the environment, for example in the bathroom or around the bed space, etc.	Enables clear access for the patient and the nurse to safely use the equipment required.
4. Wash your hands and put on an apron. Gloves should only be worn if absolutely necessary, never 'just in case'.	Wearing gloves creates a barrier between the nurse and the patient as it send signals that the nurse is undertaking 'dirty tasks'.
	Wearing an apron and gloves as part of personal protective equipment (PPE) is a standard infection-control procedure when dealing with body fluids or patients in isolation.
	Ensure your use of PPE such as gloves and disposable aprons is appropriate by considering the individual patient situation and the risk presented.
5. Ensure privacy, so close doors and curtains/blinds as necessary. If you are at a patient's bed space ensure	Patients will need to feel able to remove their clothing without being seen by others. Maintain patient privacy, dignity and comfort as required.

Step	Reason and patient-centred care considerations
you draw the curtains fully. Assist the patient to find a comfortable position and ensure they will not get cold. Do not hurry and be gentle. Only expose the area of the body you need to attend to at that particular moment.	Caring for a patient's hygiene is a personal and intimate procedure which takes time to perform with dignity. Washing areas of the body can result in cooling. Areas of skin can be very delicate.
6. As appropriate, encourage the patient to undertake as much of the process as possible.	Promotes independence.
7. Equipment used for hygiene needs, such as electric shavers, must not be shared between patients.	Reduces the risk of infection.
8. After you have completed the hygiene procedure, remove any towels that have been used to protect the patient and assist them to get into a comfortable position.	Promotes patient comfort.
9. Remove your apron and perform hand hygiene. Document in the patient's notes the care you have given and any relevant observations of pressure areas, etc.	Reduces the risk of infection. Maintains patient safety and accurate records.
10. Offer or support the patient to have a drink (so long as this is not contraindicated).	Promotes patient comfort and ensures they are well nourished and hydrated.

Evidence base: Baillie (2009); DH (2010); Dougherty and Lister (2011); Glasper et al. (2010); NICE (2012a); NMC (2007, 2015); Sargeant and Chamley (2013); Sharples (2011); WHO (2009)

Bathing a patient in bed

☑ **What is normal**

Most patients have their own hygiene practices, which may be very different from yours, so remember to ensure you are working in partnership with your patient.

Remember to constantly observe and assess the patient's skin.

☑ **Before you start**

Remember to perform the common steps (pp. 144–146).

☑ **Essential equipment**

Single-use bowl x2, warm water, towel x3, soap, incontinence pads, disposable washcloths, skin moisturizer or talc (if the patient wishes), clean clothes, nightwear or gown for the patient, clean bedlinen.

☑ **Care-setting considerations**

It is possible to bed-bath a patient in a variety of settings as long as the necessary equipment is available.

☑ **What to watch out for/action to take**

If, whilst bed-bathing a patient, any areas of skin have been observed which are abnormal, this must be reported to a relevant individual and recorded in the patient's notes.

Steps	Reason and patient-centred care considerations
1. Perform steps 1-7 of the common steps (pp. 144-146).	To prepare the patient and yourself to undertake the skill.
2. Offer assistance as required to undress the patient. Only uncover the area you are washing; the rest of the patient should remain covered by either the bed sheets or a dry towel.	Maintains patient dignity and keeps them warm.
3. Fill a bowl with fresh warm water, check the temperature	Patient safety.

Steps	Reason and patient-centred care considerations
carefully and if possible check that the patient is happy with the temperature. Change this water at any time if it becomes too cool or dirty. Always change the water after washing the perineal area and buttocks.	Reduces risk of contamination.
4. Disposable washcloths are much better than a flannel for washing patients as you can dispense of them when they have been used.	Bacteria rapidly multiply in wet, warm environments such as a flannel.
Always use new washcloths for the patient's face, torso, back and perineal area. To keep the water as clean as possible, do not put a soapy washcloth back into the water - dispose of it and use a new one.	Reduces risk of contamination.
5. Ensure the bed is at a height which is comfortable for you to work, changing this throughout the procedure as necessary.	Cares for your back.
6. Start by washing the patient's face. If possible check with the patient whether they prefer to use soap for areas of their body such as face. If you use soap, rinse it off well. Avoid getting soap in eyes.	Reduces risk of contamination.

Prevents soap left on the skin from making it dry and itchy. |
| 7. Use a clean washcloth for each part of the body. | Avoids transferring contaminants. |
| 8. Wash each area of the patient's body by wetting the washcloth and then wringing it out to prevent dripping water all over the patient. Always pat the skin thoroughly dry with a towel. If possible ask the patient whether they feel dry. | If patients are not thoroughly dried they will become cold. |

Steps	Reason and patient-centred care considerations
9. Once you have washed the patient's face, move to the arm furthest away from you. Place a towel underneath and wash the hand, then arm, then armpit using soap. Take special care to avoid any dressings or cannulae. Rinse the soap off well and dry with the towel. Repeat the process for the other arm.	Prevents dripping on areas previously washed. Reduces risk of infection.
10. Next wash the torso using soap. For female patients or men with gynecomastia, gently lift the breasts and wash underneath. Repeat this procedure with any other skin folds that may be present. Once again, be very careful not to get any dressings, drains or other lines wet. Rinse the soap off and dry the area thoroughly.	Skin under the breasts or skin folds need to be cleaned and dried to avoid fungal infections.
11. If the patient wishes, apply deodorant, moisturizer or talc. When finished cover the torso with a dry towel.	Continues the patient's normal routine. Maintains patient dignity and keeps them warm.
12. Lift the bedsheet back to expose the patient's feet and legs, but ensure you keep the genitals covered. Place a towel under the leg furthest away and wash the foot and leg with soap. Ensure you clean very gently between the toes. Rinse well. Dry thoroughly and repeat with the other foot and leg.	Prevents dripping on areas previously washed. Maintains patient dignity and keeps them warm.
13. Change the water and put on gloves if you were not already wearing them.	Potential contact with body fluids/excreta.

Steps	Reason and patient-centred care considerations
14. Ask the patient if you can wash their genitals now and obtain their consent. Some patients may wish to wash this area themselves, so offer them this opportunity.	Promotes independence and maintains dignity.
15. The genital/perineal area is very delicate and needs special care. Wash very gently with warm water alone, rinse well and pat dry. Work from the cleanest to the dirtiest area, so from the front to back (urethral to anal area). To wash an uncircumcised adult male patient you will need to gently retract the foreskin to wash the urethral meatus. Remember to gently return the foreskin after washing to prevent swelling and discomfort. If the patient is unable to do this you will need to obtain their consent and explain exactly what you are doing whilst you do it.	Reduces potential of contamination. **This would not be done with a child.**
16. If the patient has a catheter, carry out the appropriate catheter care in line with local policy.	Reduces risk of infection.
17. When clean and dry, re-cover the patient and dispose of the water and the single-use bowl. Remove your gloves and wash your hands. Reapply gloves if necessary and refill a new single-use bowl with warm water.	Maintains patient dignity and keeps them warm. Reduces risk of infection.
18. Even if the bedlinen is not wet or soiled, this is a good time to change it. If the patient is unable to move easily in the bed you will need another	Promotes patient comfort.

Steps	Reason and patient-centred care considerations
carer to assist you to change the sheets whilst the patient is still in the bed. Ensure you abide by manual handling policies and that the bed is at the correct height, and use a slide sheet if required to reposition the patient.	Cares for your back.
19. Assist the patient to roll onto their side, facing away from you and towards the other carer. Ensure the other carer is able to support the patient and the patient feels safe. Cover the patient's front with the bed sheet.	Ensures patient safety. Maintains patient dignity.
20. Roll the old sheet into the middle of the bed and place a towel behind the patient.	
21. Use soap to wash the patient's back, then rinse and dry thoroughly.	Keeps the patient warm.
22. Ask the patient's consent to wash their sacral area/ buttocks. If the patient is soiled put on gloves if you are not wearing them already. Wash, rinse and dry thoroughly. If appropriate, remove gloves, dispose of them and wash your hands.	Reduces risk of contamination.
23. Remove towel from behind patient. If sheet rolled up behind/under patient is damp or soiled, cover with an incontinence pad.	Reduces risk of contamination.
24. Tuck a clean sheet under mattress edge closest to you; smooth it over the mattress behind the patient and roll up the part which will go under the patient.	

Steps	Reason and patient-centred care considerations
25. Assist the patient to roll on to their other side; remember to tell them they will roll over a bump due to the rolled sheets. Remove old sheet and incontinence pad if appropriate. Dispose of them as per policy.	Reduces risk of infection.
26. Unroll clean sheet and tuck tightly under the mattress.	Wrinkle-free sheets promote patient comfort.
27. Assist the patient to re-dress as appropriate and move into a comfortable position.	Promotes patient comfort and dignity.
28. Finish changing the bedlinen by putting clean pillowcases on the pillows, with a clean top sheet and blankets if required.	
29. Dispose of bowl or clean with detergent and water if reusable. Store inverted to avoid dregs of water collecting in it. Dispose of/clean any other equipment as per local policy and return any of the patient's equipment to their locker. Clean the bedside table and put any belongings you moved back in their original position. If appropriate, ensure the patient can reach the nurse call bell.	Reduces risk of infection. Maintains patient safety.
30. Perform steps 8-10 of the common steps (pp. 144-146).	To ensure that: • the patient is safe, comfortable and receiving the appropriate care; • the results have been documented in the patient's records; • the equipment is clean and in working order.

Evidence base: Baillie (2009); DH (2010); Dougherty and Lister (2011); Glasper et al. (2010); NICE (2012a); NMC (2007, 2015); Sargeant and Chamley (2013)

Shaving

☑ **What is normal**

Most patients have their own hygiene practices, which may be very different from yours, so remember to ensure you are working in partnership with your patient.

☑ **Before you start**

Remember to perform the common steps (pp. 144–146).

☑ **Essential equipment**

Using an electric shaver – electric shaver, bowl, warm water, towel, mirror and moisturizer or aftershave (if the patient wishes).

Using a safety razor – safety razor, shaving foam, bowl, warm water, dry towel, mirror and moisturizer or aftershave (if the patient wishes).

☑ **Field-specific considerations**

When assisting a patient with a learning disability it may be important to ascertain what a patient's usual shaving routine is, as they may not be able to tell you.

Patients with mental health problems – who are severely depressed, for example – may not view their personal hygiene as important, so both physical and psychological support could be required.

☑ **Care-setting considerations**

Ensure patient dignity is maintained as most individuals carry out all of their hygiene practices in private.

Shaving can be undertaken in any care setting.

☑ **What to watch out for/action to take**

If you observe any skin areas that are abnormal you need to report this to a relevant individual, record it in the patient's notes and omit step 5, as this may potentially aggravate the areas.

Step	Reason and patient-centred care considerations
1. Perform steps 1-7 of the common steps (pp. 144-146).	To prepare the patient and yourself to undertake the skill.
2. Drape a towel around the patient's front.	Protects clothes.
3. Wash the patient's face and dry it thoroughly.	Cleans the area, enables observation of the skin plus any shaving preferences, such as sideburns, etc.
4. If any of the stubble is more than 1 cm or so long, use a beard-trimmer to cut this first.	Long hairs will be pulled out rather than cut by an electric shaver or safety razor.

Step		Reason and patient-centred care considerations
Electric shaver	**Safety razor**	Results in the closest, most comfortable shave and prevents skin from becoming sore.
a. Shave in the opposite direction to hair growth, making small circular motions if the patient has short stubble. For longer stubble create larger circular motions. b. Avoid repeatedly shaving the same area.	a. Apply shaving foam to the patient's face and neck. b. Pull the area you are about to shave taut – where you start is a matter of preference. c. Angle the razor to approx. 45 degrees away from the face. Using as little pressure as possible, move the razor across the skin in the direction of hair growth. d. Repeat this process once more on the same area of skin and then move to another area. e. Frequently dip the razor into the warm water. f. If there is a large amount of stubble you may need to use more than one safety razor. g. Rinse the patient's face with cool water when you have finished shaving all areas.	To remove the hair and shaving foam. To remove any excess shaving foam.
5. If the patient desires apply moisturizer or aftershave, but remember if you use aftershave to apply it sparingly, as it can sting.		Enables patient to continue their usual hygiene practices. Do not apply moisturizer or aftershave to areas of sore or broken skin.
6. Assist the patient to look at his face in the mirror to ensure they approve of the result.		Helps the patient present themselves in the manner they desire.
7. Perform steps 8-10 of the common steps (pp. 144-146).		To ensure that: • the patient is safe, comfortable and receiving the appropriate care; • the results have been documented in the patient's records; • equipment is clean and in working order.

Evidence base: Baillie (2009); DH (2010); Dougherty and Lister (2011); NICE (2012a); NMC (2007, 2015)

Teeth-cleaning

☑ **What is normal**
Most patients have their own hygiene practices, which may be very different from yours, so remember to ensure you are working in partnership with your patient.

☑ **Before you start**
Remember the 'common steps' (pp. 144–146).

☑ **Essential equipment**
Toothbrush, toothpaste, disposable cup, bowl, towel, mouthwash (if the patient wishes) and mirror.

☑ **Field-specific considerations**
When assisting a patient with a learning disability it may be important to ascertain what a patient's usual teeth-cleaning routine is, as they may not be able to tell you.

Patients with mental health problems – who are severely depressed, for example – may not view their personal hygiene as important, so both physical and psychological support could be required.

When caring for a child, encourage and assist parents or carers to be involved in hygiene care to maintain the usual routine. Supporting, educating and enabling parents or carers to continue their care within any environment is an important nursing role.

☑ **Care-setting considerations**
Ensure patient dignity is maintained, as most individuals carry out all of their hygiene practices in private.

Teeth-cleaning can be undertaken in any care setting.

☑ **What to watch out for/action to take**
Remember to constantly observe and assess the patient's tongue and oral structures. If you observe any areas that are abnormal you need to report this to a relevant individual and record it in the patient's notes.

Step	Reason and patient-centred care considerations
1. Perform steps 1-7 of the common steps (pp. 144-146).	To prepare the patient and yourself to undertake the skill.
2. Drape a towel around the patient's front.	Protects clothes.

Step	Reason and patient-centred care considerations
3. Apply a pea-sized blob of toothpaste to the toothbrush. Ask the patient to open their mouth and, holding the brush at 45 degrees, use small circular motions to brush the teeth.	Effectively cleans teeth.
4. Brush the upper teeth first, brushing all surfaces, paying extra attention to the area where the teeth and gums meet.	Particles gather between the teeth and gums.
5. When you have brushed all areas, offer the patient diluted mouthwash or water to rinse.	Removes toothpaste and particles.
6. Assist the patient to look at their teeth in the mirror to ensure they approve of the result.	Enables the patient to present themselves in the manner they desire.
7. Perform steps 8-10 of the common steps.	To ensure that: • the patient is safe, comfortable and receiving the appropriate care; • the results have been documented in the patient's records; • the equipment is clean and in working order.

Evidence base: Baillie (2009); DH (2010); Dougherty and Lister (2011); Glasper et al. (2010); NICE (2012a); NMC (2007, 2015); Sargeant and Chamley (2013)

Assisting a patient with a wash (out of bed)

☑ **What is normal**

Most patients have their own hygiene practices, which may be very different from yours, so remember to ensure you are working in partnership with your patient.

Remember to constantly observe and assess the patient's skin.

Before you start:

Remember to perform the common steps (pp. 144–146).

Essential equipment

Single-use bowl, warm water, towels, soap, incontinence pads, disposable washcloths, skin moisturizer, talc and deodorant (if the patient wishes), clean clothes, nightwear or gown for the patient.

Care setting considerations:

It is possible to assist a patient with a wash in all settings as long as the necessary equipment is available. If it is appropriate take the patient to the bathroom. If the patient is unable to leave their bed-space, clear sufficient space on their table and assist them to sit in a chair.

What to watch out for/action to take:

If whilst washing a patient any areas of skin have been observed which are abnormal this must be reported to a relevant individual and recorded in the patient's notes.

Steps	Reason and patient-centred care considerations
1. Perform steps 1-7 of the common steps (pp. 144-146).	To prepare the patient and yourself to undertake the skill.
2. Offer assistance as required to undress the patient. Only uncover the area you are washing; use towels to cover the rest of the patient.	Maintains patient dignity and keeps them warm. If you are at the patient's bed-space ensure you draw the curtains fully.
Assist the patient to find a comfortable position.	Encourage the patient to undertake as much of the process as possible to promote independence
	Sitting upright makes the process of washing easier.
3. Fill a bowl with fresh warm water, check the temperature carefully and if possible check that the patient is happy with the temperature. Change this water at any time if it becomes too cool or dirty. Always change the water after washing the perineal area and buttocks.	Patient safety. Reduces risk of contamination.
4. Disposable washcloths are much better than a flannel for washing patients as you can dispense of them when they have been used.	Bacteria rapidly multiply in wet, warm environments such as a flannel.

Steps	Reason and patient-centred care considerations
Always use a new washcloth for the patient's face, torso, back and perineal area. To keep the water as clean as possible do not put a soapy washcloth back into the water; dispose of it and use a new one.	Reduces risk of contamination.
5. Ensure the bowl and the patient are at a height which is comfortable for you to work, changing this throughout the procedure as necessary.	Cares for your back.
6. Start by washing the patient's face. If possible check with the patient whether they prefer to use soap for areas of their body such as face. If you use soap rinse it off well. Avoid getting soap in eyes.	Reduces risk of contamination. Prevents soap left on the skin from making it dry and itchy.
7. Use a clean washcloth for each part of the body.	Avoids transferring contaminants.
8. Wash each area of the patient's body by wetting the washcloth and then wringing it out to prevent dripping water all over the patient. Always pat the skin thoroughly dry with a towel. If possible ask the patient whether they feel dry.	If patients' are not through dried they will become cold.
9. Once you have washed the patient's face move to the arm furthest away from you. Wash the hand, then arm then armpit using soap. Take special care to avoid any dressings or canulae. Rinse the soap off well and dry with the towel. Repeat the process for the other arm.	Prevents dripping on areas previously washed. Reduces risk of infection.
10. Next wash the torso and back using soap. For female patients or men with gynecomastia gently lift the breasts and wash underneath. Repeat this procedure with any other skin folds that may be present. Once again be very careful not to get any dressings, drains or other lines wet. Rinse the soap off and dry the area thoroughly.	Skin under the breasts or skin folds needs to be cleaned and dried to avoid fungal infections.

Steps		Reason and patient-centred care considerations
11.	If the patient wishes apply deodorant, moisturizer or talc. When finished cover the torso and back with a dry towel.	Continues the patient's normal routine. Maintains patient dignity and keeps them warm.
12.	Expose the patient's feet and legs, but ensure you keep the genitals covered. Start with the leg furthest away and wash the foot and leg with soap. Ensure you clean very gently between the toes. Rinse well. Dry thoroughly and repeat with the other foot and leg.	Maintains patient dignity and keeps them warm.
13.	Change the water and put on gloves if you were not already wearing them.	Potential of contact with body fluids/excreta.
14.	Ask the patient if you can wash their genitals and sacral area and obtain their consent. Some patients may wish to wash this area themselves, so offer them this opportunity.	Promotes independence and maintains dignity.
15.	The genital/perineal area is very delicate and needs special care. Wash very gently with warm water alone, rinse well and pat dry. Work from the cleanest to the dirtiest area, so from the front to back (urethral to anal area). To wash an uncircumcised adult male patient you will need to gently retract the foreskin to wash the urethral meatus. Remember to gently return the foreskin after washing to prevent swelling and discomfort. If the patient is unable to do this you will need to obtain their consent and explain exactly what you are doing whilst you do it.	Reduces potential of contamination. **This would not be done with a child.**
16.	If the patient has a catheter; carry out the appropriate catheter care in line with local policy.	Reduces risk of infection.
17.	When clean and dry recover the patient and dispose of the water and the single use bowl. Remove your gloves and wash your hands. Reapply gloves if necessary and refill a new single use bowl with warm water.	Maintains patient dignity and keeps them warm. Reduces risk of infection.

Steps	Reason and patient-centred care considerations
18.	Assist the patient to re-dress as appropriate and move into a comfortable position.	Promotes patient comfort and dignity.
19.	Dispose of bowl or clean with detergent and water if reusable. Store inverted to avoid dregs of water collecting in it. Dispose of/clean any other equipment as per local policy and return any of the patient's equipment to their locker. Clean the bed-side table and put any belongs you moved back in their original position. If appropriate ensure the patient can reach the nurse call bell.	Reduces risk of infection. Maintains patient safety.
20.	Perform steps 8-10 of the common steps (pp. 144–146).	To ensure that the: • patient is safe, comfortable and receiving the appropriate care; • results have been documented in the patient's records; • equipment is clean and in working order.

Evidence base: Baillie (2009); DH (2010); Doughtery and Lister (2011); Glasper et al. (2010); NICE (2012a); NMC (2007, 2015); Sargeant and Chamley (2013)

Trimming nails

☑ What is normal
Most patients have their own hygiene practices, which may be very different from yours, so remember to ensure you are working in partnership with your patient.

Remember to constantly observe and assess the condition of the patient's nails and surrounding skin.

☑ Before you start
Remember to perform the common steps (pp. 144–146).

☑ Essential equipment
Scissors, nail clippers, nail file, soap/hand cleanser, bowl, warm water, towel, hand-lotion if the patient wishes.

☑ Care setting considerations

It is possible to trim a patient's nails in all settings as long as the necessary equipment is available.

☑ What to watch out for/action to take

If any areas of skin or any nails have been observed which are abnormal this must be reported to a relevant individual and recorded in the patient's notes.

Steps		Reason and patient-centred care considerations
1. Perform steps 1-7 of the common steps (pp. 144-146). Offer assistance as required to prepare the patient so you are able to access the nails you are going to trim. Only uncover the area you are working on. Assist the patient to find a comfortable position.		To prepare the patient and yourself to undertake the skill. Maintains patient dignity. If you are at the patient's bed-space ensure you draw the curtains fully.
2. Fill a bowl with fresh warm water, check the temperature carefully and if possible check that the patient is happy with the temperature. Change this water at any time if it becomes too cool or dirty.		Patient safety. Reduces risk of contamination.
3. Ensure the bowl and the patient are at a height which is comfortable for you to work, changing this throughout the procedure as necessary.		Cares for your back.
4. Trimming fingernails Soak the patient's hands in the water and gently clean around and underneath their nails if required.	Trimming toenails Soak the patient's feet in the water, wash their feet and gently clean around and underneath their nails if required. Check their feet for any signs of:	Reduces risk of contamination. Assess the condition of the skin and nails and ensure any potential problems are reported.

Steps		Reason and patient-centred care considerations
	Check the condition of the patient's nail beds; are there any signs of inflammation (redness) or fungus (discolouration)? If so report this to your mentor or a registered nurse.	<ul><li>redness, warmth, soreness or pain (infection)</li><li>numbness or tingling (neuropathy)</li><li>dry or cracked skin</li><li>swelling</li><li>blisters, cuts, scratches or sores</li><li>in-growing toenails, corns, calluses</li><li>toenail fungus (discolouration).</li></ul>If you find any of the above report it to your mentor or a registered nurse.	
5.	Dry the patient's hands and nails carefully.	Dry the patient's feet very carefully, especially between their toes.	To promote comfort and prevent the patient from feeling cold.
6.	Trim one nail at a time. If after trimming any nails have a rough edge you will need to wait until the nail is properly dry and then file it smooth.	Trim one nail at a time. Cut the nail straight across. Do not cut down into the corners, you should still be able to see the white tip at the top edge. If after trimming any of the nails still have a rough edge wait until the nail is properly dry and then file it smooth.	To ensure nails are not cut too short and are smooth so they do not catch on clothing or scratch skin.
7.	Apply hand-lotion if the patient wishes.	If the patient desires you can apply lotion to the top and bottom of their feet, but not between the toes.	

Steps	Reason and patient-centred care considerations
8. Dispose of bowl or clean with detergent and water if reusable. Store inverted to avoid dregs of water collecting in it. Dispose of/ clean any other equipment as per local policy and return any of the patient's equipment to their locker. If appropriate clean the bed-side table and put any belongs you moved back in their original position. Ensure the patient can reach the nurse call bell.	Reduces risk of infection. Maintains patient safety.
9. Perform steps 8-10 of the common steps (pp. 144-146).	To ensure that the: • patient is safe, comfortable and receiving the appropriate care; • results have been documented in the patient's records; • equipment is clean and in working order.

Evidence base: Baillie (2009); DH (2010), Doughtery and Lister (2011); Glasper et al. (2010); NICE (2012a); NMC (2007, 2015); Sargeant and Chamley (2013)

Washing a patient's hair in bed

☑ **What is normal**

Most patients have their own hygiene practices, which may be very different from yours, so remember to ensure you are working in partnership with your patient.

Remember to constantly observe and assess the condition of patient's hair and skin on their scalp.

☑ **Before you start**

Remember to perform the common steps (pp. 144–146).

☑ Essential equipment

Bed hair-rinser, towel x3, large incontinence pads, patient's shampoo, brush and comb, bowl x2, warm water, jug, mirror and any other hair product the patient uses.

☑ Care setting considerations

It is possible to wash a patient's hair in bed in any setting as long as the necessary equipment is available.

☑ What to watch out for/action to take

If whilst washing a patient's hair any areas of skin have been observed which are abnormal this must be reported to a relevant individual and recorded in the patient's notes.

Steps	Reason and patient-centred care considerations
1. Perform steps 1-7 of the common steps (pp. 144-146).	To prepare the patient and yourself to undertake the skill.
2. Offer assistance as required to prepare the patient. Draw the curtains fully around the patient's bed-space if appropriate.	Maintains patient dignity and keeps them warm.
Clear sufficient space around the patient's bed, pull it out so you can easily access the head end, and ensure you reapply the brakes.	To enable you to move freely in the bed space.
Wrap a towel around the patient's shoulders.	To stop them from getting wet.
3. Make sure that the patient is comfortable whilst you are undertaking the next step, 'preparing the bed and bed-space', moving them following safe patient moving principles.	To promote patient comfort. Preparing the bed-space effectively is most important, as otherwise the procedure will not go smoothly.
4. Lay the patient and the bed flat, so you can either fold the bed's headboard down, as some can be used as a shelf at the top of the bed, or remove it completely.	Ensure that the patient is able to tolerate lying flat. To effectively prepare the bed space.
If the headboard cannot be used as a shelf move the patient's bed table to this position, as this is where the bed hair-rinser will go.	To enable equipment to be at hand when you need it.
Position another table as close to the top of the bed as possible and place the jug and a bowl of clean warm water on this table.	

Steps	Reason and patient-centred care considerations
5. Place a towel on the bed head or table and place the bed hair-rinser on top. Position the spout so it hangs over the side; place a large incontinence pad on the floor underneath this with an empty bowl on top to collect the waste water.	To prevent water from escaping and wetting the floor.
6. Assist or move the patient to a comfortable position where their head is laying in the bed hair-rinser.	To ensure the patient is in the correct position to have their hair washed.
7. Use the jug to wet the patient's hair with the warm water in the bowl. Check that the patient is happy with the temperature of the water and protect their eyes and ears. Do not hurry and be gentle.	To promote patient comfort whilst washing their hair.
8. Put a small amount of shampoo on the palm of your hand and rub it in to the patient's hair and scalp with circular movements. Rinse the hair with warm water, repeating as often as necessary until all of the lather from the shampoo has been washed away. Repeat the shampooing and rinsing stages until the hair is clean.	
9. Wrap a clean towel around the patient's hair and assist or move their head out of the bed hair-rinser.	To remove equipment no longer required.
10. Ensure the patient is in a comfortable position and ask them how they wish their hair to be styled. If local policy allows use a hairdryer to dry their hair.	To promote patient comfort.
11. Assist the patient to look at their hair in a mirror to ensure they approve of the result. Remove the towel from the patient's shoulders and ensure they are in a comfortable position.	To ensure the patient is happy with the end result of their hair washing and drying.

Steps	Reason and patient-centred care considerations
12. Dispose of bowls or clean with detergent and water if reusable. Store inverted to avoid dregs of water collecting in it. Dispose of/clean any other equipment as per local policy and return any of the patient's equipment to their locker. Clean the bed-side table and put any belongs you moved back in their original position. Ensure the patient can reach the nurse call bell.	Reduces risk of infection. Maintains patient safety.
13. Perform steps 8–10 of the common steps (pp. 144–146).	To ensure that the: • patient is safe, comfortable and receiving the appropriate care; • results have been documented in the patient's records; • equipment is clean and in working order.

Evidence base: Baillie (2009); DH (2010); Doughtery and Lister (2011); Glasper et al. (2010); NICE (2012a); NMC (2007, 2015); Sargeant and Chamley (2013)

PERFORMING LAST OFFICES

JEAN SHAPCOTT

Performing Last Offices

☑ **Before you start**
Remember to ensure that the death of the patient has been confirmed, that you know whether there is going to be a post-mortem and that, if relevant/appropriate, the family have been offered the opportunity to assist in performing Last Offices.

☑ **Essential equipment**
All settings
Disposable aprons and gloves; bowl of warm water; patient's own toilet articles; disposable washcloths; towels x 2; patient's own razor/disposable razor (if male); comb and equipment for nail care; equipment for mouth care, including care of patient's dentures; plastic bags for clinical and domestic waste; container for expressed urine; clean linen; any documentation required by law or local policy; shroud or culturally appropriate clothing or patient's own clothes if requested by family.

Community setting
Toe tag (for identification)

Hospital setting
Linen skip for soiled linen, identification bands x2, valuables/property book, bag(s) for patient's own property

If required
Gauze, dressings and tapes to cover wounds, IV sites, etc.; caps/spigots for urinary catheters, drains, etc. if they are to be left in situ

For children

Card/envelope to keep a lock of hair, washable paint and card for hand/foot-prints, toy, etc. that family may wish to leave with the child after procedure is completed

☑ **Care-setting considerations**

Last Offices can be performed in both hospital and community care settings.

Steps	Reason and patient-centred care considerations
1. Gather the equipment required. Ensure these are clean as appropriate.	To be fully prepared and organized. Reduces the chance of infection and maintains patient and nurse safety.
2. Ensure privacy, so close doors and curtains/blinds as necessary. If you are at a patient's bed space ensure you draw the curtains fully.	Maintain patient privacy and dignity as required.
3. Tidy the bed space; turn off monitoring equipment. If possible remove equipment from the bedside.	To normalize the environment for relatives or carers and provide access to safely perform the procedure.
4. Wash your hands and put on an apron. Wear apron throughout procedure and gloves whenever appropriate.	Personal protective equipment (PPE) must be worn when performing Last Offices to protect yourself and other patients from the risk of infection. However, this needs to be done in a way that maintains dignity and respect. If family members are present, be especially sensitive to their views relating to this; consider how they might feel if gloves are worn when, for example, washing the face of their loved one.
5. If the patient was being nursed on a pressure-relieving mattress or device, consult manufacturer's guidance before turning it off.	If the mattress is allowed to deflate too quickly, it may pose a moving and handling challenge when performing Last Offices.

Steps	Reason and patient-centred care considerations
6.	Lay the patient on their back with their limbs as straight as possible whilst adhering to local moving and handling policy.	It will not be possible to do this at a later stage. Stiff, flexed limbs can be difficult for mortuary staff to manage and can cause additional distress to family members or carers who wish to view the body. However, if it is not possible to straighten the patient's body or limbs, do not use force; it can be corrected later by the undertaker.
7.	Close the patient's eyes by applying light pressure to the eyelids for approximately 30 seconds. If this is unsuccessful, moistened cotton wool can be used to maintain the position of the eyelids until they remain closed. Some policies suggest the use of tape to keep eyelids closed.	To maintain the patient's dignity, for aesthetic reasons and to minimize distress of relatives who may wish to view the body. Only tape that does not mark the skin on removal should be used, and this should not be done to the eyelids of a child.
8.	If it is certain that there is not to be a post-mortem, all drains, cannulae, catheters, etc. can be removed and disposed of appropriately. Gauze dressings may be applied over entry sites. If there is to be a post-mortem, leave all drains, cannulae, catheters, etc. in situ, disconnect as close to the body as possible and spigot as necessary.	To leave the deceased in as natural a state as possible for family members who may wish to view the body. To prepare the body for burial or cremation. To comply with legal requirements and facilitate investigation into the cause of death.
9.	Any wounds should be covered with a clean absorbent dressing and secured with an occlusive dressing or waterproof tape. Stitches and clips should be left intact.	The dressing will absorb leakage from the wound site and prevent oozing of blood or serous fluid.

Steps	Reason and patient-centred care considerations
10. Drain the patient's bladder by applying gentle pressure over the lower abdomen.	To ensure the bladder contains minimal volume of urine and prevent leakage of body fluids.
11. Leakage of body fluids from the oral cavity can be contained by the use of suction. Incontinence pads should be used to contain leakage from the vagina and bowel. Stomas should be covered with a new bag. The packing of orifices can cause damage to the body and should not be done.	Leaking orifices pose a health hazard to staff coming into contact with the patient's body. Ensuring that the body is clean demonstrates continuing respect for the patient's dignity.
12. Wash the patient in the same way you would when undertaking a bed bath, unless requested not to do so for cultural or religious reasons or the family or carer's preference. If family members wish to assist, facilitate their participation.	For aesthetic and hygiene purposes. This is also both a mark of respect and a point of closure in the relationship between nurse and patient. The involvement of family members in washing the body is an expression of respect and affection as well as part of the process of adjusting to their loss and expressing their grief.
13. Mouth and teeth should be cleaned using foam sticks or a toothbrush. If the patient normally wore dentures, clean them and place them in their mouth. Apply petroleum jelly or equivalent to dry lips.	The patient's teeth and mouth are cleaned to remove debris for aesthetic and hygiene purposes. If dentures are not re-inserted into the mouth the patient may appear very different to the way they appeared in life.
14. *Death in hospital* Ensure all the patient's property is gathered together and placed in a clearly labelled bag. In the presence of another nurse, remove all jewellery from the body unless the family request otherwise. Record the jewellery and other valuables, storing them in accordance with local policy.	To respect relatives' wishes and comply with both legal requirements and cultural practices. Sensitivity is required when clothing is soiled and you should not assume that the family wish to keep it - always ask.

Steps	Reason and patient-centred care considerations
Avoid using the names of precious metals or gems when recording jewellery - instead use terms such as 'white metal' and 'green stone'.	To ensure items are accurately described, as it can be very difficult to tell precious metals or stones from imitation ones.
Any jewellery left on the body should be secured with tape.	To ensure it remains with the patient.
All jewellery remaining on the body should be documented on the Notification of Death form.	To provide a formal record of what has been left on the patient.
Death at home	
Work closely with the patient's family to ensure their wishes and those of the deceased are followed.	
15. Dress the patient in a shroud or other clothing as required by cultural tradition or requested by family members. Children are not normally dressed in a shroud and parents often have specific requests as to what they should wear.	For aesthetic reasons for family members or others who may wish to view the body, to comply with religious or cultural requirements and to meet the needs of the family members or carers.
Remember that at this point there may still be some leakage from body orifices, so it is not appropriate to dress the body in clothing that the family may wish them to wear for burial or cremation.	
16. *Death in hospital* Ensure two fully completed patient identification bands are attached to the patient - one on the wrist and one on the ankle. Complete all necessary documentation, such as Notification of Death cards, and tape such card to the shroud or clothing.	To ensure accurate and easy identification of the patient's body in the mortuary.

Steps	Reason and patient-centred care considerations
Death at home Ensure that a toe tag (or equivalent) is attached to the patient and that all necessary documentation is completed and ready to accompany the body.	
17. Wrap the patient's body in a sheet, ensuring that all the limbs are held securely in position and the face and feet are covered. For a child, ensure any toy that the parents have requested should accompany the body is secured within the sheet.	To avoid possible damage to the patient's body during transfer and prevent distress to colleagues (such as porters in the hospital setting).
18. Secure the sheet with tape.	Pins should not be used as they present a health and safety hazard.
19. If required by local policy or for infection-control purposes, place the body in a body bag and ensure that information regarding any known infectious disease is clearly documented and visible.	Placing the body in a body bag is advised for all notifiable diseases and some other infectious diseases (such as HIV), and a label clearly identifying the infection must be attached to the patient's body. Whilst it is true that certain additional precautions are required when performing Last Offices on a patient with a disease known to be infectious who has died, the body poses no greater infection risk than it did whenthat patient was alive. The application of standard infection-control practices must therefore be continued when handling the body of the deceased.
20. Tidy up the area, complete any further documentation and clean any reusable equipment.	To ensure that: • the patient's records are updated; • equipment is clean and in working order.

Evidence base: Dougherty and Lister (2011); Green and Green (2006); HSAC (2003); NMC (2015)

APPENDIX 1

COMMONLY USED MEDICATION AND SIDE EFFECTS

You should also check the cautions, contraindications and dose. Continue to build up your list of known medication following the information below.

Cardiovascular system		
Name	**Indications**	**Side Effects**
Amlodipine	Hypertension, prophylaxis of angina	Abdominal pain, nausea, palpitations, flushing, oedema, headache, dizziness, sleep disturbances, fatigue
Aspirin	Secondary prevention of thrombotic cerebrovascular or cardiovascular disease	Bronchospasm, gastro-intestinal irritation, gastrointestinal haemorrhage
Atenolol	Hypertension, angina, arrhythmias	Gastrointestinal disturbances, bradycardia, heart failure, hypotension
Atorvastatin	hypercholesterolemia	Myalgia, myopathy, gastro-intestinal disturbances, sleep disturbances, headache, dizziness

Cardiovascular system

Name	Indications	Side Effects
Digoxin	Heart failure, supraventricular arrhythmias	Nausea, vomiting, diarrhoea, arrhythmias, dizziness, blurred vision, rash
Diltiazem	Prophylaxis and treatment of angina, hypertension	Bradycardia, palpitations, dizziness, hypotension, malaise, headache, hot flushes, oedema
Glyceryl trinitrate	Angina	Postural hypotension, tachycardia, throbbing headache, dizziness
Isosorbide mononitrate	Prophylaxis of angina, adjunct in congestive cardiac failure	Postural hypotension, tachycardia, throbbing headache, dizziness
Lisinopril	Hypertension and heart failure	Hypotension, renal impairment, persistent dry cough, rash
Nicorandil	Prophylaxis and treatment of stable angina	Nausea, vomiting, rectal bleeding, flushing, increase in heart rate, dizziness, headache
Nifedipine	Prophylaxis of angina, hypertension	Gastro-intestinal disturbances, hypotension, oedema, vasodilatation, palpitations, headache, dizziness, lethargy
Pravastatin	hypercholesterolemia	Myalgia, myopathy, gastro-intestinal disturbances, sleep disturbances, headache, dizziness
Ramipril	Hypertension, symptomatic heart failure	Hypotension, renal impairment, persistent dry cough
Simvastatin	hypercholesterolemia	Myalgia, myopathy, gastro-intestinal disturbances, sleep disturbances, headache, dizziness
Spironolactone	Oedema and ascities	Gastro-intestinal disturbances, malaise, confusion, drowsiness, dizziness

Central nervous system

Name	Indications	Side Effects
Carbamazepine	Focal and secondary generalized tonic-clonic seizures, trigeminal neuralgia	Headache, ataxia, drowsiness, nausea, vomiting, blurred vision
Citalopram	Depressive illness, panic disorder	Nausea, vomiting, dyspepsia, abdominal pain, diarrhoea, constipation, anorexia, rash
Co-codamol	Mild to moderate pain	Nausea, vomiting, constipation, dry mouth, biliary spasm, respiratory depression, hypotension, muscle rigidity
Diazepam	Short-term use in anxiety and insomnia, adjunct in acute alcoholic withdrawal	Drowsiness and light headedness the next day, confusion, ataxia, amnesia, dependence, muscle weakness
Fluoxetine	Major depression, bulimia nervosa, obsessive compulsive disorder	Diarrhoea, dysphagia, vasodilation, hypotension, flushing, palpitations
Lorazepam	Status epilepticus, febrile convulsions	Drowsiness and light headedness the next day, confusion, ataxia, amnesia, dependence, muscle weakness
Methadone	Severe pain, cough in terminal disease, adjunct in treatment of opioid dependence	Nausea, vomiting, constipation, dry mouth, biliary spasm,
Morphine sulphate	Severe pain	Nausea, vomiting, constipation, dry mouth, biliary spasm
Paracetamol	Mild to moderate pain, pyrexia	Side effects rare
Paroxetine	Major depression, obsessive-compulsive disorder, panic disorder, post-traumatic stress disorder	Nausea, vomiting, dyspepsia, abdominal pain, diarrhoea, constipation, anorexia, rash

Central nervous system

Name	Indications	Side Effects
Risperidone	Schizophrenia and other psychoses	Tremor, dystonia, restlessness, sexual dysfunction, tachycardia, arrhythmias, hypotension
Sertraline	Depressive illness, obsessive-compulsive disorder, panic disorder	Nausea, vomiting, dyspepsia, abdominal pain, diarrhoea, constipation, anorexia, rash
Temazepam	Insomnia	Drowsiness and light headedness, confusion, ataxia
Tramadol	Moderate to severe pain	Nausea, vomiting, constipation, dry mouth, biliary spasm, diarrhoea, retching, fatigue
Venlafaxine	Major depression, generalized anxiety disorder	Constipation, nausea, anorexia, weight changes, vomiting hypertension, palpitations
Zopiclone	Insomnia	Taste disturbance, nausea, vomiting, dizziness, drowsiness, dry mouth, headache

Endocrine system

Name	Indications	Side Effects
Gliclazide	Used in diabetes	Gastro-intestinal disturbances
Levothyroxine	hypothyroidism	Diarrhoea, vomiting, angina pain, arrhythmias, palpitations, tachycardia, tremor, restlessness
Metformin	Diabetes mellitus	Anorexia, nausea, vomiting, diarrhoea, abdominal pain, taste disturbance

Gastro-intestinal system

Name	Indications	Side Effects
Lactulose	constipation	Nausea, vomiting, flatulence, cramps and abdominal discomfort
Lansoprazole	Gastric ulcer, eradication of Helicobacter pylori	Nausea, vomiting, abdominal pain, flatulence, diarrhoea, constipation and headache
Omeprazole	Gastric and duodenal ulcers	Gastro-intestinal disturbances, headache, agitation, impotence
Ranitidine	Benign gastric and duodenal ulceration, dyspepsia	Diarrhoea, headache, dizziness
Senna	Constipation	Abdominal cramp

Infections

Name	Indications	Side Effects
Amoxicillin	Urinary tract infections, sinusitis, bronchitis	Nausea, vomiting, diarrhoea, rashes
Cefalexin	Broad-spectrum antibiotic which is used to treat septicaemia, pneumonia, meningitis, biliary-tract infections, peritonitis and urinary-tract infections	Diarrhoea, nausea and vomiting, abdominal discomfort, headache, rashes
Erythromycin	Oral infections, campylobacter enteritis, syphilis, respiratory tract infections, skin infections	Nausea, vomiting, abdominal discomfort, diarrhoea
Flucloxacillin	Otitis externa, adjunct in pneumonia, impetigo, cellulites	Gastro-intestinal disturbances
Metronidazole	Clostridium difficile infections, leg ulcers and pressure sores, bacteria vaginosis, ulcerative gingivitis, oral infections	Gastro-intestinal disturbances, taste disturbances, furred tongue, oral mucositis, anorexia

Musculoskeletal and joint disease

Name	Indications	Side Effects
Ibuprofen	Pain and inflammation in rheumatic disease, mild to moderate pain, migraine, dental pain	Gastro-intestinal disturbances including discomfort, nausea, diarrhoea, occasionally bleeding and ulceration.
Naproxen	Pain and inflammation in rheumatic disease, dysmenorrhoea, acute gout	Gastro-intestinal disturbances including discomfort, nausea, diarrhoea, occasionally bleeding and ulceration.

Nutrition and blood

Name	Indications	Side Effects
Ferrous sulphate	Iron-deficiency anaemia	Gastro-intestinal irritation, nausea, epigastric pain, diarrhoea, constipation
Folic acid	Anaemia	Gastro-intestinal disturbances

Respiratory System

Name	Indications	Side Effects
Salbutamol	Asthma, conditions associated with reversible airways obstruction	Fine tremor, nervous tension, headache, muscle cramps, palpitations

Source: www.medicinescomplete.com/mc/bnf/current

APPENDIX 2

NORMAL LABORATORY VALUES

ADULT	CHILD			
Haematology:	RBC	Male	Female	μ/L = mm^3
Red Blood Cells (RBC) Men 4.5-6.5 x 10^{12}/L Women 3.9-5.6 x 10^{12}/L	6 months	4.2-5.5	3.4-5.4 x	10^6 / μ/L
	6 months-2 years	4.1-5.0	4.1-4.9 x	10^6/ μ/L
	2-12 years	4.0-4.9	4.0-4.9 x	10^6 / μ/L
Haemoglobin (Hb) Men 135- 175 g/L Women 115-155 g/L	12-18 years	42-53	40-49	
White Blood Cells (WBC) Men 3.7-9.5 x 10^9/L Women 3.9-11.1 x 10^9/L	Hb	Male	Female	
	Newborn	14.7-18.6	12.7-18.3g/dL	
	6 months-2 years	10.3-12.4	10.4-12.4g/dL	
	2-6 years	10.5-12.7	10.7-12.7g/dL	
	6-12 years	11.0-13.3	10.9-13.3g/dL	
	12-18 years	11.5-14.8	11.2-13.6g/dL	
Platelets Men 150-400 x 10^9/L Women 150-400 x 10^9/L	WBC			
	Newborn	6.8-13.3	8.0-14.3 x 10^3 / μml/L	
	2 years	6.2-14.5	6.4-15.0 x 103 / μml/L	
Coagulation/INR	6months-2 years	6.2-14.5	6.4-15.0 x 10^3 / μml/L	
INR range 2-3 (in some cases a range of 3-4.5 is acceptable)	2-6 years	5.3-11.5	5.3-11.5 x 10^3 / μml/L	

ADULT	CHILD		
	6-12 years	4.4-10.5	4.7-10.3 x 10^3 / μml/L
	12-18 years	4.5-10.0	4.8-10.1 x 10^3 / μml/L
Biochemistry:	**Platelets**		
	Newborn	164-351	234-346 x 10^3 / μl/L
Sodium 135-145 mmol/L	1-2 months	275-567	295-615 x 10^3 / μl/L
	2-6 months	275-566	288-598 x 10^3 / μl/L
Potassium 3.5-5.2 mmol/L	6 months- 2 years	219-452	229-465 x 10^3 / μl/L
Urea 2.6-6.5 mmol/L	2-6 years	204-405	204-402 x 10^3 / μl/L
	6-12 years	194-364	183-369 x 10^3 / μl/L
	12-18 years	165-332	185-335 x 10^3 / μl/L
Creatinine 55-105 μmol/L	**Sodium**		
	Newborn 133-146 mmol/L		
	Children 135-145 mmol/L		
Calcium 2.2-2.6 mmol/L	**Potassium**		
	Premature Newborn 4.5-7.2 mmol/L		
	Full term Newborn 3.7-5.2 mmol/L		
	Children 3.5-5.8 mmol/L		
	Urea		
	1-3 years 1.8-6.0 mmol/L		
	4-13 years 2.5-6.0 mmol/L		
	14-19 years 2.9-7.5 mmol/L		

ADULT	CHILD		
C reactive protein (CRP) <10mg/L	**Creatinine**	**Male**	**Female**
	1-3 days	17.7-88.4	17.7-88.4 µmol/L
	1 year	17.7-53.0	17.7-44.2 µmol/L
	2-3 years	17.7-61.9	26.5-53.0 µmol/L
	4-7 years	17.7-70.7	17.7-61.9 µmol/L
	8-10 years	26.5-79.6	26.5-70.7 µmol/L
	11-12 years	26.5-88.4	26.5-79.6 µmol/L
	13-17 years	26.5-106.1	26.5-97.2 µmol/L
	18-20 years	44.2-115	26.5-97.2 µmol/L
Albumin 35-50g/L	**Calcium** Premature Newborn (first week) 1.7-2.3 mmol/L		
	Full term Newborn (first week) 2.0-2.5 mmol/L		
	Children 2.2-2.6 mmol/L		
Bilirubin (Total)< 17 ⇌mol/L	**Albumin** Newborn 2.6-3.6 g/dL		
	1-3 years 3.4-4.2 g/dL		
	4-6 years 3.5-5.2 g/dL		
	7-9 years 3.7-5.6 g/dL		
	10-19 years 3.7-5.6g/dL		
	Bilirubin Neonates (Total) < 10 µmol/L		

APPENDIX 3

SKILLS MAPPED TO NMC ESSENTIAL SKILLS CLUSTERS

Chapter	Skill	Relevant NMC Essential Skills Clusters
Infection Prevention and Control	Hand-washing	Cluster: Care, compassion and communication
	Using hand sanitizer	1 - 7. All first and second progression points.
	When to remove your gloves and why	Cluster: Infection prevention and control
		21. By the first progression point - 1.
		22. By the first progression point - 1.
Clinical Measurement	Common steps for all clinical measurement	Cluster: Care, compassion and communication
	Counting a respiratory rate	1 - 7. All first and second progression points.
	Measuring SpO$_2$	Cluster: Organizational aspects of care
	Measuring a pulse rate	9. By the first progression point - 1.
	Automated blood pressure measurement	9. By the second progression point - 2, 6, 7, 8, 9, 10, 11.
	Manual blood pressure measurement	
	Measuring capillary refill time	15. By the first progression point - 1.
	Measuring body temperature	20. By the first progression point - 1.
	Blood glucose monitoring	Cluster: Infection prevention and control
		21. By the first progression point - 1.
		22. By the first progression point - 1.
		22. By the second progression point - 3, 4, 5, 6.

Chapter	Skill	Relevant NMC Essential Skills Clusters
Pain Management	Undertaking a pain assessment	<u>Cluster: Nutrition and fluid management</u> 27. By the second progression point - 2. 28. By the second progression point - 1. 29. By the second progression point - 1, 2. <u>Cluster: Care, compassion and communication</u> 1 - 7. All first and second progression points. <u>Cluster: Organizational aspects of care</u> 9. By the first progression point - 1. 15. By the first progression point - 1. <u>Cluster: Infection prevention and control</u> 21. By the first progression point - 1.
Aseptic Technique and Specimen Collection	Principles of asepsis Common steps for the collection of all types of specimen Taking a wound swab Collecting a faeces specimen Collecting a urine specimen Collecting a sputum sample Taking a nasal swab Taking a throat swab	<u>Cluster: Care, compassion and communication</u> 1 - 7. All first and second progression points. <u>Cluster: Organizational aspects of care</u> 15. By the first progression point - 1. <u>Cluster: Infection prevention and control</u> 21. By the first progression point - 1. 21. By the second progression point - 2, 3, 4, 5. 22. By the first progression point - 1. 23. By the second progression point - 2, 3, 4, 5, 6

Chapter	Skill	Relevant NMC Essential Skills Clusters
Skin Integrity	Principles of caring for a patient with a wound	Cluster: Care, compassion and communication
	Pressure ulcers - quick reference guide	1 - 7. All first and second progression points.
		Cluster: Organizational aspects of care
		15. By the first progression point - 1.
		Cluster: Infection prevention and control
		21. By the first progression point - 1.
		22. By the first progression point - 1.
		Cluster: Nutrition and fluid management
		27. By the second progression point - 1, 2, 3.
Safer Handling of People	Efficient movement principles	Cluster: Care, compassion and communication
	A safe way of working when moving a patient	1 - 7. All first and second progression points.
		Cluster: Organizational aspects of care
		15. By first progression point - 1.
		17. By first progression point - 1, 2.
		20. By first progression point - 1.
		Cluster: Infection prevention and control
		21. By first progression point - 1.
		22. By first progression point - 1.

Chapter	Skill	Relevant NMC Essential Skills Clusters
First Aid	The recovery position	Cluster: Care, compassion and communication
	ABCDE summary actions	1 - 7. All first and second progression points.
	Management of choking	Cluster: Organizational aspects of care
	AVPU assessment	9. By the first progression point - 1.
		15. By the first progression point - 1.
		Cluster: Infection prevention and control
		21. By the first progression point - 1.
		22. By the first progression point - 1.
Medicines Administration	Administering medication (oral or topical route)	Cluster: Care, compassion and communication
	Administering a subcutaneous injection	1 - 7. All first and second progression points.
	Administering an intramuscular injection	Cluster: Organizational aspects of care
		10. By the second progression point - 1, 2.
		15. By the first progression point - 1.
		Cluster: Infection prevention and control
		21. By the first progression point - 1.
		22. By the first progression point - 1.
		22. By the second progression point - 2, 3, 4,5,6.
		Cluster: Medicines management
		33. By the first progression point - 1.

Chapter	Skill	Relevant NMC Essential Skills Clusters
		34. By the second progression point – 1, 2, 3.
		36. By the second progression point – 1.
		37. By the second progression point – 1.
		38. By the second progression point – 1, 2, 3.
		40. By the second progression point – 1.
		41. By the second progression point – 1.
Assisting Patients with their Nutritional Needs	Common steps for all nutrition-related skills	Cluster: Care, compassion and communication
		1 – 7. All first and second progression points.
	Weighing a patient	Cluster: Organizational aspects of care
	Assisting a patient to eat and drink	9. By the second progression point – 2, 3, 4, 5.
	Passing a nasogastric tube	15. By the first progression point – 1.
	Confirmation of position of a nasogastric tube	Cluster: Infection prevention and control
	Maintaining a nasogastric tube	21. By the first progression point – 1.
	Caring for a PEG (pertcutaneous endoscopic gastronomy)	22. By the first progression point – 1.
	Stoma care	Cluster: Nutrition and fluid management
	Peripheral vascular cannula care	27. By the second progression point – 1, 2, 3, 4, 5.

Chapter	Skill	Relevant NMC Essential Skills Clusters
		28. By the second progression point - 1, 2, 3.
		29. By the second progression point - 1, 2, 3, 4.
		30. By the first progression point - 1, 2.
		30. By the second progression point - 3, 4.
		31. By the second progression point - 1, 2.
Assisting Patients with their Elimination Needs	Common steps for all elimination-related skills	Cluster: Care, compassion and communication
	Assessing bowel function	1 - 7. All first and second progression points.
	Assisting a patient to use a bedpan, urinal or commode	Cluster: Organizational aspects of care
		10. By the second progression point - 1, 2.
	Performing catheter care	15. By the first progression point - 1.
	Emptying a patient's catheter bag	20. By the first progression point - 1.
	Urinalysis	Cluster: Infection prevention and control
		21. By the first progression point - 1.
		22. By the first progression point - 1.
		22. By the second progression point - 2, 3, 4, 5, 6.
		26. By the second progression point - 1, 2, 3.

Chapter	Skill	Relevant NMC Essential Skills Clusters
Assisting Patients with their Hygiene Needs	Common steps for all hygiene procedures	Cluster: Care, compassion and communication
	Bathing a patient in bed	1 - 7. All first and second progression points.
	Shaving	Cluster: Organizational aspects of care
	Teeth-cleaning	10. By the second progression point - 1.
	Assisting a patient with a wash (out of bed)	15. By the first progression point - 1.
	Trimming nails	Cluster: Infection prevention and control
	Washing a patient's hair in bed	21. By the first progression point - 1.
		22. By the first progression point - 1.
Last Offices	Performing Last Offices	Cluster: Care, compassion and communication
		1 - 7. All first and second progression points.
		Cluster: Organizational aspects of care
		15. By the first progression point - 1.
		Cluster: Infection prevention and control
		21. By the first progression point - 1.
		22. By the first progression point - 1.

APPENDIX 4

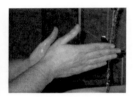

1. Wash palm to plan

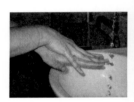

2. Rub back of both hands

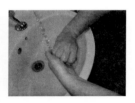

3. Rub back of fingers interlaced

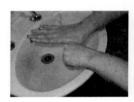

4. Wash both thumbs

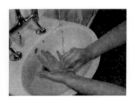

5. Rub palms with fingertips

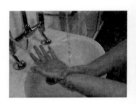

6. Wash wrists

Hand-washing technique

(Adapted from Ayliffe, 1978)

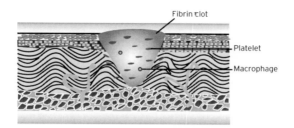

Haemostasis

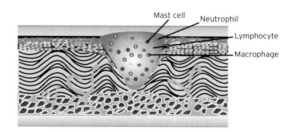

Inflammation

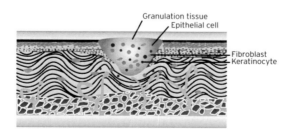

Proliferation

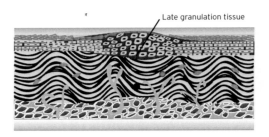
Late granulation tissue

Maturation

The 4 stages of wound healing

REFERENCES

Advanced Life Support (ALS) (2011) *Resuscitation Council* (UK) 6th ed. London.

Braden, B.J. (1997) 'Risk assessment in pressure ulcer prevention', in D. Krasner and D. Kane (eds), *Chronic Wound Care*. Wayne, PA: Health Management Publications.

Baillie, L. (2009) *Developing Practical Adult Nursing Skills*, 3rd ed. London: Hodder Arnold.

Ballentyne, M. and Ness, V. (2009) 'Eliminating', in C. Docherty and J. McCallum (eds), *Foundation Clinical Nursing Skills*. Oxford: Oxford University Press. pp. 275–307.

British Hypertension Society (2009) *Blood Pressure Measurement*. Available at: www.bhsoc.org/ latest-guidelines/how-to-measure-blood-pressure (accessed 18 February 2015).

British National Formulary (2014) *British National Formulary*, 68th ed. London: BMJ Publishing Group Ltd and Royal Pharmaceutical Society.

British Thoracic Society (2008) 'Guideline for emergency oxygen use in adult patients', *Thorax*; *BMJI*, 63 (Suppl 6): vi1–vi73.

Caton-Richards, M. (2010) 'Assessing the neurological status of patients with head injuries', *Emergency Nurse*, 17(10): 2831.

Clancy, J. and McVicar, A. (2009) *Physiology and Anatomy for Nurses and Healthcare Practitioners: A Homeostatic Approach*, 3rd ed. London: Hodder Arnold.

Cocoman A. and Murray J. (2007) 'To swab or not to swab?', *WIN*, 15 (8).

Cocoman A. and Murray J. (2008) 'Intramuscular injections: A review of best practice for mental health nurses', *Journal of Psychiatric and Mental Health Nursing*, 15: 424–434.

Dawes, E., Lloyd, H. and Durham, L. (2007) 'Monitoring and recording patient's neurological observations', *Nursing Standard*, 22(10): 40–45.

Department of Health (2010) *Essence of Care Benchmarks for Personal Hygiene*. London: DH.

Dougherty, L. and Lister, S. (2011) *The Royal Marsden Hospital Manual of Clinical Nursing Procedures*, 8th ed. Oxford: Wiley-Blackwell.

European Pressure Ulcer Advisory panel (EPUAP) (2014) *Prevention and Treatment of Pressure Ulcers: Quick Reference Guide*. Available at: www.epuap. org/wp-content/uploads/2010/10/Quick-Reference-Guide-DIGITAL-NPUAP-EPUAP_PPPIA_16Oct2014.pdf (accessed 12 March 2015).

Glasper, A., Aylott, M. and Battrick, C. (2010) *Developing Practical Skills for Nursing Children and Young People*. London: Hodder Arnold.

Green, J. and Green, M. (2006) *Dealing with Death: A Handbook of Practices, Procedures and Law*. London: Jessica Kingsley Publishers.

Hall, C. (2002) *An Evaluation of Nurse Preparation and Practice in Administering Medicine to Children*. PhD thesis, School of Education, University of Nottingham.

Health and Safety Advisory Committee (HSAC) (2003) *Safe Working and the Prevention of Infection in the Mortuary and Post-mortem Room*. London: Health and Safety Advisory Committee/HSE.

Health and Safety Executive (HSE) (2000) *The Management of Health and Safety at Work Regulations 1999*. Sudbury, Suffolk: Health and Safety Executive Books.

Health and Safety Executive (HSE) (2004) *Manual Handling. Manual Handling Operations Regulations 1992 (as amended). Guidance on Regulations L23*, 3rd ed. Sudbury, Suffolk: Health and Safety Executive Books.

The Health and Safety (Sharp Instruments in Healthcare) Regulations 2013. Available at: www.legislation.gov.uk/uksi/2013/645/made (accessed 25 March 2015).

Health Protection Scotland (2012) *Targeted Literature Review: What are the Key Infection Prevention and Control Recommendations to Inform a Peripheral Vascular Catheter (PVC) Maintenance Care Quality Improvement Tool?* [Online]. Available at: www.documents.hps.scot.nhs.uk/hai/infection-control/evidence-for-care-bundles/literature-reviews/pvc-mainte nance-review-v2.pdf (accessed 5 January 2015).

Health Protection Agency (2012a) *Investigation of Skin, Superficial and Non-surgical Wound Swabs*. UK Standards for Microbiology Investigations. Bacteriology. B11 issue no 5.1. London: Health Protection Agency.

Health Protection Agency (2012b) *Investigation of Bronchoalveolar Lavage, Sputum and Associated Specimens*. UK Standards for Microbiology Investigations. Bacteriology. B57 issue no 2.4. London: Health Protection Agency.

Health Protection Agency (2014) *Investigation of Bronchoalveolar Lavage, Sputum and Associated Specimens*. UK Standards for Microbiology Investigations. Bacteriology. B57 issue no 2.5. London: Public Health England. Available at: www.gov.uk/government/uploads/system/uploads/attachment_data/file/343994/B_57i2.5.pdf (accessed 3 March 2015).

Hunter, D. (2012) 'Conditions affecting the foreskin', *Nursing Standard*, 26(37): 35–9.

Jevon, P. (2010) 'How to ensure patient observations lead to effective management of patients with pyrexia', *Nursing Times*, 106 (1): 16–18.

Leaver, R.B. (2007) 'The evidence for urethral meatal cleansing', *Nursing Standard*, 21 (41): 39–42.

Loveday, H., Wilson, J., Pratt, R., Golsorkhi, M., Tingle, A., Bak, A., Browne, J., Prieto, J. and Wilcox, M. (2013) 'EPIC 3, national evidence-based guidelines for preventing healthcare-associated infections in NHS hospitals in England' *Journal of Hospital Infection*, 86S1: S1–S70. Available at: www.his.org.uk/files/3113/8693/4808/epic3_National_Evidence-Based-Guidelines_for_Prevention-HCAI_in_NHSE.pdf (accessed 24 March 2015)

Marieb, N.E. (2013) *Human Anatomy and Physiology*. Boston MA: Pearson.

McCallum, L. and Higgins, D. (2012) 'Care of peripheral venous cannula sites', *Nursing Times,* 108 (34/35): 12–15.

McCallum, L. and Higgins, D. (2012) 'Measuring body temperature', *Nursing Times*, 108 (45): 20–2.

Mulryan, C. (2011) *Acute Illness Management*. London: SAGE.

National Institute for Health and Care Excellence (NICE) (2003) *Infection Control: Prevention of Healthcare-associated Infection in Primary and Community Care.* London: NICE.

National Institute for Health and Care Excellence (NICE) (2006) *Nutrition Support in Adults. Oral Nutrition Support, Enteral Tube Feeding and Parenteral Nutrition. Clinical Guideline 32.* London: NICE.

National Institute for Health and Care Excellence (NICE) (2011a) *Knee Pain Assessment.* Available at: http://cks.nice.org.uk/knee-pain-assessment (accessed 18 February 2015).

National Institute for Health and Care Excellence (NICE) (2012a) *Prevention and Control of Healthcare-Associated Infections in Primary and Community Care. Clinical Guideline 139.* London: NICE. Available at: http://guideline.nice.org.uk/CG139 (accessed 24 March 2015).

National Institute for Health and Care Excellence (NICE) (2012b) *Quality Standard for Nutrition Support in Adults.* London: NICE.

National Institute for Health and Care Excellence (2013) *Neuropathic Pain – The Pharmacological Management of Neuropathic Pain in Adults in Non-specialist Settings.* Available at: http://guidance.nice.org.uk/CG/Wave0/629 (accessed 18 February 2015).

National Institute for Health and Care Excellence (NICE) (2014a) *Acutely Ill Patients in Hospital.* Available at: http://pathways.nice.org.uk/pathways/acutely-ill-patients-in-hospital (accessed 30 October 2014).

National Institute for Health and Care Excellence (NICE) (2014b) *Pressure Ulcers: Prevention and Management of Pressure Ulcers. Clinical Guideline 179.*

London: NICE. Available at: www.nice.org.uk/guidance/cg179/resources/guidance-pressure-ulcers-prevention-and-management-of-pressure-ulcers-pdf (accessed 2 March 2015).

National Patient Safety Agency (2011) *Reducing the Harm Caused by Misplaced Nasogastric Feeding Tubes in Adults, Children and Infants.* Available at: www.nrls.npsa.nhs.uk/alerts/?entryid45=129640&q=0%C2%ACnasogastric+feeding+tubes%C2%AC

National Patient Safety Agency (2012) *Harm from Flushing of Nasogastric Tubes before Confirmation of Placement.* Available at: www.nrls.npsa.nhs.uk/resources/?entryid45=133441&q=0%C2%ACnasogastric+tubes%C2%AC (accessed 24 March 2015).

National Prescribing Centre (NPC) (n.d.) *A Guide to Good Practice in the Management of Controlled Drugs in Primary Care (England).* Available at: www.npc.nhs.uk/controlled_drugs/resources/controlled_drugs_third_edition.pdf (accessed 24 March 2015).

NHS Greater Glasgow and Clyde (2012) *Standard Operating Procedure (SOP): Insertion & Maintenance of Indwelling Urinary Catheters.* Available at: http://library.nhsgg.org.uk/mediaAssets/Infection%20Control/SOP%20Urinary%20Catheters%20V3%20-%2026.09.12.pdf (accessed 18 February 2015).

Nursing and Midwifery Council (2007, ratified 2008) *Standards and Guidance for Medicines Management.* London: NMC.

Nursing and Midwifery Council (2009) *Record Keeping.* London: Nursing and Midwifery Council. Available at: www.nmc-uk.org/Documents/NMC-Publications/NMC-Record-Keeping-Guidance.pdf (accessed 24 March 2015).

Nursing and Midwifery Council (2010a) *Standards and Guidance for the Delivery of Pre-registration Nursing Education.* London: NMC.

Nursing and Midwifery Council (2010b) *Standards for Medicines Management.* London: NMC.

Nursing and Midwifery Council (2015) *The Code: Professional Standards of Practice and Behaviour in Nursing and Midwifery.* London: NMC.

Oxford University Hospitals NHS Trust (2013) *Oxford Pelvic Floor Service: Obstructive Defaecation. Patient Advice and Information Leaflet on the Management of Obstructive Defaecation.* Available at: www. ouh.nhs.uk/patient-guide/leaflets/files%5C130124obstructivedefaecation.pdf (accessed 18 February 2015).

Piper, B., Langemo, D. and Cuddigan, J. (2009) 'Pressure ulcer pain', *Ostomy Wound Management*, Feb: 16–31.

Polak, F. (2011) 'Mechanics and human movement', in J. Smith (ed.), *The Guide to the Handling of People: A Systems Approach*, 6th ed. Teddington: Backcare. pp. 53–61.

Public Health England (2014a) *Investigation of Skin, Superficial and Non-surgical Wound Swabs.* UK Standards for Microbiology Investigations.

Bacteriology. B11 issue no 5.2. London: Public Health England. Available at: https://www.gov.uk/government/uploads/system/uploads/attachment_ data/file/391745/B_11i5.2.pdf (accessed 3 March 2015).

Public Health England (2014b) *Investigation of Faecal Specimens for Enteric Pathogens*. UK Standards for Microbiology Investigations. Bacteriology. B30 issue no 8.1. London: Public Health England. Available at: www.gov.uk/gov ernment/uploads/system/uploads/attachment_data/file/343955/B_30i8.1.pdf (accessed 3 March 2015).

Public Health England (2014c) *Investigation of Urine*. UK Standards for Microbiology Investigations. Bacteriology. B41 issue no 7.2. London: Public Health England. Available at: www.gov.uk/government/uploads/ system/uploads/attachment_data/file/343969/B_41i7.2.pdf (accessed 3 March 2015).

Public Health England (2014d) *Investigation of Throat Swabs*. UK Standards for Microbiology Investigations. Bacteriology. B9 issue no 8.3. London: Public Health England. Available at: www.gov.uk/government/uploads/ system/uploads/attachment_data/file/356254/B_9i8.3.pdf (accessed 3 March 2015).

Public Health (2014e) *Investigation of Bronchoalveolar Lavage, Sputum and Associated Specimens*. UK Standards for Microbiology Investigations. Bacteriology B57 issue no. 2.5. Available at: www.gov.uk/government/ uploads/system/uploads/attachment_data/file/343994/B_57i2.5.pdf (accessed 25 March 2015).

Public Health England (2015) Investigation of nasal samples. Bacteriology B, issue 7.1. London: Public Health England. Available at: /www.gov.uk/ government/uploads/system/uploads/attachment_data/file/394716/ B_5i7.1.pdf (accessed 25 March 2015).

Resuscitation Council (UK) (2010) *Resuscitation Guidelines 2010*. London. Resuscitation Council (UK).

Royal College of Nursing (RCN) (2011a) *Sharps Safety RCN Guidance to Support the Implementation of EU Directive 2010/32/EU Prevention of Sharps Injuries in the Health Care Sector*. London: RCN. Available at: www. rcn.org.uk/_data/assets/pdf_file/0008/418490 (accessed 24 March 2015).

Royal College of Nursing (2011b) *Nutrition Now: Enhancing Nutritional Care*. Available at: www.rcn.org.uk/__data/assets/pdf_file/0006/187989/003284. pdf (accessed 24 February 2015).

Royal College of Nursing (2012) *Tools of the Trade*. London: RCN.

Sargeant, S. and Chamley, C. (2013) 'Oral health assessment and mouthcare for children and young people receiving palliative care', *Nursing Children and Young People*, 25(3): 30–3.

Schoonhoven, L., Haalboom, R., Buskens, E. et al (2002) 'Prognostic ability of risk assessment scales', *EPUAP Review*, 4 (1): 17–18.

Scottish Intercollegiate Guidelines Network (2012) *SIGN Guideline 119: Management of Patients with Stroke: Identification and Management of Dysphagia (2013).* Available at: www.sign.ac.uk/guidelines/fulltext/119/section6.html (accessed 12 March 2014).

Sharples, K. (2011) *Successful Practice Learning for Nursing Students*, 2nd ed. London: SAGE.

SIGN (2001) *Guideline 119: Management of Patients with Stroke: Identification and Management of Dysphagia.* Available at: www.sign.ac.uk/guidelines/fulltext/119/section6.html (accessed 18 February 2015).

Simons, S. and Remington, R. (2013) 'The Percutaneous Endoscopic Gastronomy Tube: A Nurses Guide to PEG Tubes', *Medsurg Nursing*, 22 (2): 77–83.

Smith, G. (2012) *ALERT. Acute Life-threatening Events, Recognition and Treatment, A Multi-professional Course in Care of the Acutely Ill Patient*, 3rd ed. Portsmouth: Institute of Medicine. Available at: www.alert-course.com (accessed 18 February 2015).

Smith, J. (ed.) (2011) *The Guide to the Handling of People: A Systems Approach*, 6th ed. Teddington: Backcare.

Smith, J. and Roberts, R. (2011) *Vital Signs for Nurses: An Introduction to Clinical Observations.* Oxford: Wiley-Blackwell.

Taylor, S.J. Allan, K. McWilliam, H. and Toher, D. (2014) 'Nasogastric tube depth: the "NEX" guideline is incorrect', *British Journal of Nursing*, 23: 12.

Trott, A.T. (2005) *Wounds and Lacerations: Emergency Care and Closure*, 3rd ed. London: Elsevier.

Waterhouse, C. (2009) 'The use of painful stimulus in relation to Glasgow Coma Scale observations', *British Journal of Neuroscience Nursing*, 5 (5): 209–214.

Waterlow J.A. (2005) *Pressure Area Prevention Manual*. Taunton: J.A. Waterlow.

Westbrook, J., Woods, A., Rob, M., Dunsmuir W. and Day, R. (2010) 'Association of interruptions with an increased risk and severity of medication administration errors', *Arch Intern Med.*, 170 (8): 683–690.

WHO (2009) *WHO Guidelines on Hand Hygiene in Health Care.* Available at: http://whqlibdoc.who.int/publications/2009/9789241597906_eng.pdf (accessed 24 March 2014).

WHO (2014) *Giving Safe Injections. A Guide for Nurses and Others Who Give Injections.* Available at: www.who.int/occupational_health/activities/1bestprac.pdf (accessed 5 June 2014).

Willock, J., Baharestani, M.M. and Anthony, D. (2009) 'The development of the Glamorgan paediatric pressure ulcer risk assessment scale', *Journal of Wound Care*, 18 (1): 17–21.